PREVENTING HEART DISEASE
Exercising for A Healthy Heart

The best way to improve your overall health is through cardio-vascular fitness. The American Heart Association advises regular exercise as a positive measure for preventing cardiovascular disease. Studies at Stanford University School of Medicine have shown that those who exercise regularly are not only significantly less prone to heart attacks, but the effect of a heart attack is far less severe than on those who do not exercise regularly.

This is your personal handbook for achieving cardiovascular fitness. It will help you to develop, evaluate and tailormake your personal exercise programme for total health and longevity based on your age, life-style, sex and personal exercise or sport preference. Included in the book are concise instructions, illustrations and schedules on types and amounts of exercise, tips on nutrition, guidance on pre-exercise medical checkup and how to avoid problems of over exercise.

If you are concerned about losing a few kilos, improving muscle tone, lowering the chance of heart disease or just looking good, this is the book for you.

PAUL VODAK is an physiologist at the Stanford Heart Disease Prevention Program in Palo Alto, California, and a member of the American College of Sports Medicine. He has been a special consultant and a clinic supervisor at the U.S. National Athletic Health Institute, Los Angeles, providing fitness evaluation and counselling for business executives and professional athletes.

D1293927

EXERCISING

FOR A

HEALTHY HEART

PAUL VODAK
Exercise Physiologist
Stanford Heart Disease Prevention Program

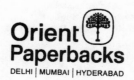

Orient
Paperbacks

DELHI | MUMBAI | HYDERABAD

www.orientpaperbacks.com

ISBN 13: 978-81-222-0163-5
ISBN 10: 81-222-0163-6

1st Published 1995
6th Printing 2006

Preventing Heart Disease: Exercising for a Healthy Heart
(Originally Published as *Exercise: The Why & The How*)

Published in arrangement with
Bull Publishing Company, USA

Cover design by Vision Studio

Published by
Orient Paperbacks
(A Division of Vision Books Pvt. Ltd.)
5A/8 Ansari Road, New Delhi-110 002

Printed in India at
Ravindra Printing Press, Delhi-110 006

Contents

1
Why Exercise?

Towards Physical Fitness

The world is currently experiencing an unprecedented obsession with physical fitness. The interest has definitely passed the 'fad' stage and is evidenced by staggering growth in all areas of sport and recreation. Apparently the age of the 'arm-chair athlete' is slowly giving way to the age of the 'sports' participant'. According to a Gallup poll taken in the US recently, nearly half of all adult Americans—47%—reported regular participation in some form of physical exercise. This is twice the percentage reported two decades ago. This trend, by all available accounts, has accelerated further during the last decade and a half.

The sport of running is probably the most visible example of the fitness craze. A friend named Peter mentioned, how, in 1960, he and a handful of men ran 7 km. through downtown San Francisco in the annual Bay-to-Breakers Race. After several years the number of entries reached five hundred, and many of Peter's friends elected not to run because the course was becoming too crowded. I first ran in the Bay-to-Breakers in 1977. Upon reaching the starting area and thinking of Peter's comments, I had to chuckle—waiting for the gun were over twelve thousand men, women and children!

Although running has obviously become the recognised symbol of physical fitness, by no means is it the most popular sport. Sindlinger's Economic Service (SES), a marketing and opinion research firm in USA, reports that there are almost four times as many swimmers as runners in America today. Number two on their list of favourite participant sports is tennis. SES claims that 35 million players are wandering around looking for someone to 'ace'. The exact number is hard to verify but one thing is sure: you have to get out of bed much earlier every morning to find an empty court.

Most recently racquetball has captured great interest, earning itself the undisputed title of the fastest growing sport. This exciting game is played indoors and is like a fusion of handball and squash. The main reason for its tremendous appeal is its simplicity. Even a first-time novice can hit the ball against the front wall and immediately experience the thrill of competitive action. Estimations of the number of racquetball enthusiasts range from three to five million, but the rate of growth is limited only by the shortage of playing facilities.

All other areas of the sport and recreation industry are recording similar growth statistics. People today are spending more than ever before for home conditioning equipment like stationary bicycles, treadmills, barbells, slant boards, and vibrating belts. Enrolment in local health clubs—which emphasize weight lifting, calisthenics and sauna baths is up by 25% from a year ago. Old 'traditional' sports such as golf, bowling and softball are thriving. Newly popularised sports like soccer, cross-country skiing and backpacking find people eager to spend time and money to participate on a regular basis.

What is the underlying reason for this national trend towards physical fitness? Public surveys identify not one, but many motivating factors. Some are common to many people, while others are more personal and often difficult to identify. Your motivations may fall into both categories.

As you read through the next few pages, make a mental note of those beneficial aspects you identify with. The more reasons you have for exercising, the greater will be your motivation to start, restart or maintain a regular programme of exercise.

Just for Fun

The public's conception of exercise has changed dramatically over the past 20 years. The identification is no longer one of drudgery in dismal gymnasiums! Being athletic is now a status symbol. Women who used to avoid physical education class in high school are now bragging about their two-handed backhands. Men who could never find the time to wash the car or cut the lawn are now running for a half an hour every day of the week.

The 'Pepsi Generation' is a commercial slogan, but it is easy to see why the image appeals. People today have more money and leisure time than ever before, and want to put more 'living' into their lives. Participation in sport and recreational activities is the answer for those who seek more than sedentary spectating.

Physical activity or 'play' is a primitive drive we all possess, and when fulfilled, leads to sensations of vitality and exhilaration. A well-hit forehand, a ski run through freshly fallen snow or a steady three mile run can all provide exciting moments of physical joy. That sensation of 'letting go' and exerting your muscles makes you feel young and energetic.

Sports offer additional opportunities for social interaction. Formal competition at several skill levels, and often at varying age levels, can easily be found through local sport clubs, city recreation departments or amateur athletic organisations. It is not uncommon

PER CENT OF U. S. ADULTS
WHO PARTICIPATED IN SELECTED ACTIVITIES

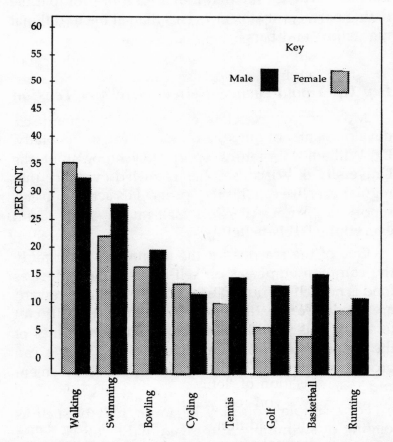

Figure 1. Per cent of persons 20 years of age and over who participated in selected exercises and sport. Source: Advance data from *Vital and Health Statistics* of the National Center for Health Statistics, USA.

to find couples planning their vacation or weekends around sporting events, such as tennis tournaments, running meets or skiing weekends. Many unmarried men and women say that they find more compatible dating partners at athletic events than at the traditional nightclubs and bars.

Pep Up Your Psyche: Relieve Stress & Tension

Most people associate exercise with just muscle development, not thinking of what it can do mentally. Dr William Morgan, a sports psychologist at the University of Wisconsin, has recorded evidence that regular exercise can 'lift the spirits'. His active subjects report a better physical self-image and claim everything 'feels better'.

One of the reasons for the mental lift is certainly the common emphasis on self-improvement. Just as food is needed for our bodies, achievement and reward are needed for healthy egos. Sometimes it is difficult to satisfy this 'mental hunger' within the confines of the domestic environment. Exercise and sports can provide a unique opportunity for finding achievement and reward.

For example, you may begin an activity such as jogging or swimming at the minimal levels of half a km or three pool lengths, and feel exhausted at the end of each session. With a few weeks of regular participation, however, you can see and feel tremendous improvement in your capacity. Your jog becomes a strong and steady 3 km. run or now, you swim ten pool lengths and climb out unwinded.

Another way exercise improves mental fitness is by helping people cope with the stress in their lives. Stress creates internal feelings of anxiety and muscular tension. Learning how to relax affected muscles is one of the important prerequisites for reducing stress. People have been reaching for tranquilizers to deal with stressful times; but now there is scientific evidence that regular exercise can be more powerful than drugs.

Dr Herbert deVries, professor of gerentology at the University of Southern California, measured muscle tension at two different times in stress-affected adults: once, after ingestion of a common tranquilizer, and then, after a brisk 75-minute walk. Interestingly, there was no change in muscle tension after taking the pill, but the short walk produced a 23% reduction. Dr deVries also points out that tranquilizers can impair muscle coordination and reaction time; in contrast, exercise leads to muscle tone and strength.

These changes in mental attitude are certainly healthy personally, but they can mean more than a better individual state of mind—for instance, they can lead to a happier and more effective work experience. In 1972, the National Aeronautics and Space Administration discovered that a formal employee exercise programme could improve work performance. Those employees who participated regularly claimed that they could work harder both mentally and physically, and they enjoyed their jobs more. The normal work routine seemed to be less boring. They reported greater stamina, increased energy and a more positive work attitude.

Shaping Up

We are all concerned about our personal appearance. For some, this means losing a few kilograms of body fat to achieve an ideal weight. For others, it means improving muscle size or tone for better body shape. Exercise plays an important role in both, but unfortunately, it is an area clouded by myth and falsehood.

For example, most people believe that overweight is related only to excessive food intake, and that exercise has little effect on weight control. However, a study comparing living habits of obese and non-obese teenage girls during 3 months at summer camp, proved that inactivity can be a main cause of overweight. There was no difference in the caloric intake of the two sets of girls. But a hidden camera showed the obese teenagers spending most of their time standing or sitting, while their normal-weight counterparts were running and jumping. Such studies have led many health experts to believe that the slow weight gain most people experience with age (creeping obesity), is not due to increased food intake, but rather, to a reduction in physical activity.

Another popular notion is that increased exercise

stimulates appetite, and that the additional food eaten will offset any progress made. Dr Jean Mayer, a nationally recognised nutritionist, tested this theory. In a famous study, he showed that men with sedentary desk jobs actually ate more food and had greater body weight compared to men with light to moderately active jobs. Dr Mayer claims that moderate exercise makes the appetite centre in the brain more sensitive to the body's real need for food.

All health professionals will agree that the best weight-loss method is a combined programme of moderate diet and moderate exercise. Attempting to lose weight rapidly by fasting, can lead to problems. Most of the early weight loss in crash programmes represents body water, which is quickly regained once normal eating habits resume. Prolonged semi-starvation diets will deprive the body of important proteins, vitamins and minerals leaving the dieter weak and irritable. On the other hand, a combination of daily exercise and moderate reduction in caloric intake leaves room for needed nutrients and still allows you to lose significant amounts of body fat.

Physical appearance is also dependent upon the quality of underlying muscle quality, but for different reasons. Men desire enlarged protruding muscles which represent strength and power. Women, on the other hand, are biologically unable to increase muscle bulk (which is fine with them), and exercise to improve muscle tone. They are looking for a flat abdomen and firm thighs.

All vigorous exercises will improve muscle definition and muscle tone. The simple 'burning of calories' will reduce surface fat, exposing the hard muscle tissue. However, for men who want muscle bulk, or for men and women who want increased strength, a special type of exercise is needed, called Progressive Resistance Training (PRT). The most common form of PRT is weightlifting, with a progression every two weeks to greater amounts of weight. The length of the programme will depend upon individual condition and the amount of strength desired.

Developing Healthy Habits

Daily living habits are among the most important determinents of health. Periodic visits to the doctor are beneficial for the detection and treatment of disease, but personal behaviour is usually the only source of prevention. A 5-year study of seven thousand adults showed that health and life expectancy are significantly related to

1   Three meals a day, at regular times with no snacks.
2   Breakfast every day.
3   Moderate exercise two or three times a week.
4   Adequate sleep (7 or 8 hours a night).
5   No smoking.
6   Moderate weight.
7   No alcohol (or only in moderation).

To summarise the study results, a 45-year-old man with 0-3 of these characteristics has a remaining life expectancy of 22 years (age 67), while one with 6-7 has a life expectancy of 33 years (to age 78). In other words, 11 years could be added to life expectancy by making simple changes in daily living habits. Moreover, with improved health, the quality of life during those years is greatly enhanced.

Other medical studies have focused concern on two other aspects of personal behaviour that affect physical health: diet and stress. It appears that people who constantly eat high-fat foods, sugared sweets or high-salt foods have a greater risk of experiencing any one of several health problems. And stress (often the result of high-pressure occupations and/or major changes in life situations) can render one more susceptible, not only to cardiovascular disease, but to infectious diseases as well.

Scientists have not identified the perfect lifestyle that will ensure a disease-free existence, but enough information is available to enable significant changes in the odds in favour of good personal health, and one does not have to become a 'health nut'. Modest changes in daily habits, sustained throughout life, have a much better effect than drastic changes initiated on a whim. A prescription of behaviour change costs nothing, and there is no risk involved in the treatment. If anything, you will look and feel better and have more energy. Literally, by adopting the modest habits of a healthy lifestyle, you have nothing to lose and everything to gain.

Preventing Heart Disease

Exercise is one of the important positive* 'health habits', having its greatest impact on the prevention of cardiovascular disease. This chronic disease of the heart and blood vessels is a major health problem in most parts of the world today, accounting for 50% of all deaths.

Studies have shown that regular physical activity can reduce your chances of a heart attack. Moreover, if you sustain a heart attack, the effect will probably be less severe if you are physically fit. The American Heart Association takes the position that it is 'prudent' to exercise regularly. And now, life insurance companies are offering reduced premiums for those people who remain active.

Dr Ralph Paffenbarger jr. professor at Stanford University School of Medicine, has looked closely at the relationship between exercise and heart disease. In one study of seventeen thousand men aged 35-75, he discovered significantly fewer heart attacks among those who regularly engaged in such vigorous sports as running, tennis, swimming, and handball. Moreover, this trend extended to those with elevated exposure to other heart disease risk factors. Dr Paffenbarger acknowledges that exercise does not guarantee freedom from heart disease, but he calculates that if all the study subjects had been physically active, there would have been 25% fewer heart attacks.

---

* Negative habits include smoking, excessive alcohol intake and excessive caloric intake.

The exact mechanism by which physical activity 'protects' the heart still eludes scientists. They do know, however, that heart attacks can occur if the heart muscle does not receive sufficient oxygen-rich blood from the small coronary arteries—when these arteries become 'clogged' with cholesterol deposits. Regular exercise may help. Research with animals has shown increased coronary blood flow with exercise, through increased size or number of arteries; humans may benefit in a similar way.

More recent research suggests that the way cholesterol is carried in the blood may be important. For many years, biochemists have known that cholesterol is carried by two different proteins: HDL or High Density Lipoprotein and LDL or Low Density Lipoprotein. An interesting evaluation of data from the Framingham Heart Study has recently revealed an inverse relationship between the incidence of heart disease and the blood level of HDL. That is, the higher the HDL level in the blood, the better off the people seemed to be. Scientists now hypothesize that LDL is the 'bad' cholesterol that clogs the small coronary arteries, and that HDL is the 'good' cholesterol that may actually keep the arteries clean.

The search is now on for anything that will increase blood levels of HDL, but, to date, there has been only one method that produces a significant and reliable change—exercise. Dr Wood from the Stanford Heart Disease Prevention Programme compared the HDL levels of a group of avid male and female runners (age 35-59) with values in normal sedentary adults. The runners had a much higher HDL level: 34% for the women and 48% for the men. This is exciting evidence and could very well explain why people who exercise have healthier hearts.

It is important to realise that these potential cardiovascular benefits cannot be stored. Dr Paffenbarger verified this by comparing the health of two groups: one of ex-college athletes and the other of men who were inactive in college. The athletes who discontinued exercise after college had the normal high percentage of heart attacks, whereas the inactive college men who later formed regular exercise habits experienced significantly fewer heart attacks. This and other similar studies suggest that physical activity of 5, 10, or 15 years ago does not reduce the present risk of heart disease.

Therefore, exercise habits should be maintained year-round, year after year, if you want to keep the benefits. To some this may sound like an impossible task, with personal effort far outweighing possible reward. But once a regular pattern of exercise is established, activity becomes easy and natural. In fact, many active people are uncomfortable when they don't maintain their regular level of exercise.

The secret is to find one sport that you really enjoy and will concentrate on; but then have two or three others you occasionally use for diversity. The following chapters contain specific information to help you achieve this goal. A variety of sports are discussed, all of which are known to provide cardiovascular benefits. You may want to explore all of them or you may already have a favourite. No matter! The important thing is that you EXERCISE—and above all, have fun!

SUMMING UP

Almost half of the adults in America report that they exercise on a regular basis. Popular sports are as numerous and diversified as the motivating factors behind them. 'Having fun' is obviously a main reason, but people also feel better after exercise—and they certainly enjoy losing body fat and improving muscle strength and tone. While exercise is only one positive health behaviour among many, it appears to have significant effects on lowering risk of heart disease. Health benefits cannot be stored however, so it is important that exercise become a lifelong habit.

2

Exercises:
What Kind and How Much

Everyone wants to get the most for their money and effort, and so when the fitness bug bites, the logical question arises: 'What is the best kind of exercise for me?'

The answer really depends upon your individual objectives. If you want muscle strength, weightlifting is the optimal form of exercise. For those concerned about body flexibility—yoga exercises or stretch calisthenics are the answer. However, improving general personal health through weight control and cardiovascular fitness, can only be achieved with certain endurance or high-energy activities—and these will be the main focus of this book.

Fitness experts agree that general physical health is best improved with endurance activities that require stamina or 'good wind'. Moreover, activities that rely upon lower body muscles, such as brisk walking, running, jumping, and cycling are superior to those like push ups or weightlifting involving only small upper body muscles. Even though the sensation of effort may be equivalent, activities that utilise the large muscles of the legs require greater energy (burn more calories), which is the critical factor for a good, healthy workout.

Health professionals used to believe that exercises such as running—involving continuous muscular action, were the only ones that produced significant fitness results. Now, with new research, it appears that many discontinuous sports such as tennis and basketball can offer similar health benefits if they are played vigorously by skilled people.

As you can see, there is no one 'best' exercise. Many of the popular sports that qualify as good exercises are presented and discussed in Chapter 5. The large selection offers plenty of room for individual preference, and 'exercise' can become play instead of the drudgery that so many of us were conditioned to associating with it.

It will not be necessary to discuss every effective sport, so long as you can understand the specific components that make up good exercise: intensity, duration, and frequency. With this information, you can analyse any sport or exercise and evaluate its fitness qualities; you can find an activity that makes it 'play' for you.

INTENSITY: SELECTING THE RIGHT EXERCISES

After stamina and energy burning, the most important quality of exercise is the intensity of action. Exactly what is meant by exercise intensity? The simplest way to think of it is to equate it with the sensation of effort. Running uphill to catch a bus is certainly more intense than walking a dog around the block—you can feel the difference in effort.

But sports scientists need an objective measure of exercise intensity, and they get it with the heart rate. The leg muscles can sustain physical work only if there is an adequate supply of oxygen-rich blood. The heart responds to this demand by beating faster and circulating more fresh blood. As the intensity of exercise increases, more blood-oxygen is needed by the working muscles, so the heart rate increases. There is a linear relationship between the heart rate and exercise intensity. This means that you have a low heart rate only when resting, which increases proportionately with increasing exercise intensity up to your 'maximal heart rate'. From now on, exercise intensity will be identified as a percentage of maximum heart rate (%MHR).

The fitness benefits of exercise are closely related to its intensity. Research studies have shown that 70% MHR is the general training threshold, in the sense that those who exercise at heart rates less than 70% MHR, generally, do not improve their cardiovascular fitness. Interestingly, most people instinctively like

RELATIONSHIP BETWEEN HEART RATE
AND EXERCISE INTENSITY

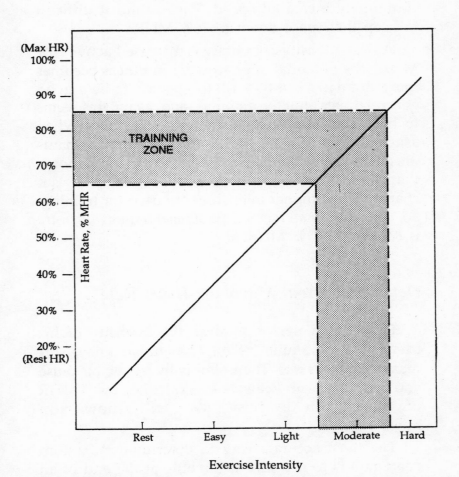

Exercise Intensity

Figure 2. Linear relationship between heart rate and exercise intensity. Intensity ratings are based on subjective feelings after 3-5 minutes of continuous exercise. Training heart rate zone is identified as 70-85% of maximum heart rate.

to exercise at 75-85% MHR. During one study, participants were asked to run at 70% MHR, but they continually increased speed. They found it difficult to keep their pace down to 70% MHR.

As the intensity of exercise is increased above 70% MHR, the potential improvement in fitness becomes more dramatic, but 85% MHR appears to be a good general upper limit for training—and, again, this seems to be a comfortable level for many people. (When asked to run at 90% MHR, the study participants unconsciously slowed down.) Also, research has shown that the incidence of muscle and bone injuries rises sharply when higher intensities are used for training. So, considering all factors, *the optimal training intensity is between 70-85% MHR.*

Determining Your Maximum Heart Rate

How can a person analyse the intensity of his exercise programme? First, he must know his maximum heart rate. Then, simply by feeling his pulse and counting heart beats, he can calculate the %MHR of any given exercise. We will show you how.

The most accurate way to determine maximum heart rate is to measure it directly, at the end of an 'all-out' muscular effort lasting 2-3 minutes. However, this special exercise stress test can be dangerous (and should be performed under a doctor's supervision, unless you know you are already in excellent shape). There is an alternative, of simply using a table which gives you an estimate on the basis of your age group; it is accurate enough for general purposes.

Scientists discovered that MHR normally declines with age: a young child can elevate heart rate to in excess of 200 beats per minute (BPM), whereas a 60-year-old peaks around 160 BPM. This relationship to age is quite consistent, and a fairly accurate estimation of anyone's maximum heart rate can be made by using the equation:

Maximum Heart Rate = 220 − Age

Figure 3 summarises heart rate information for various age groups and outlines the proper training zone. As an example, a 45-year-old person would have an estimated maximum heart rate of 175 BPM. The lower level of training intensity (70% MHR) would be 123 BPM.

Of course if you have taken a direct measure of your MHR, use that and ignore the age column in calculating your training intensity.

How To Measure Heart Rate/Pulse

To take your pulse, use a watch that shows seconds.

1. Hold the wrist with your right hand (see illus. on p. 31) and move the first two fingers of your right hand until you can feel the pulse just under your

MAXIMUM HEART RATE
AND TRAINING HEART RATE ZONE

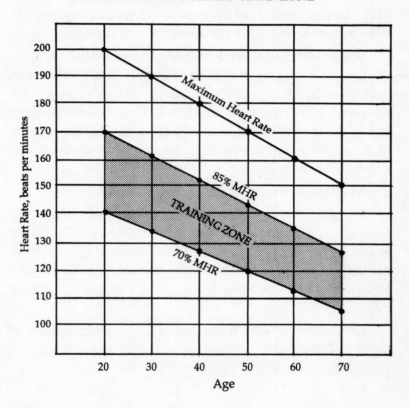

Figure 3. Estimated maximum heart rate and calculated training heart rates (70-85% MHR) for various ages. If actual MHR is known, calculate 70-85% of real value to determine training heart rate zone.

thumb on the left wrist.

2. Count the number of beats that occur during a sixty second interval.

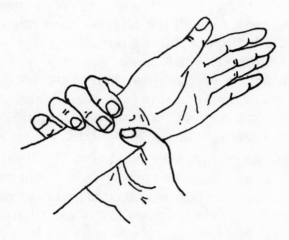

To get the 'resting pulse', you should do this first thing in the morning, while sitting in a relaxed position.

When exercising, it is important to count your pulse immediately upon stopping because heart rate begins to slow down very quickly. (It should only take 5 seconds to stop and find your pulse, and the 10 additional seconds to count your heart rate; so the whole procedure will be completed in 15 seconds.)

Adjusting Your Exercise Plan

The value of any exercise for you can now be analysed simply by comparing the heart rate you achieve during that exercise, to your prescribed training heart rates. If the exercise heart rate is lower than 70% MHR, the activity is of little value, and you should either exercise more vigorously or change activities. If the exercise heart rate is greater than 85% MHR, you may be pushing too hard. Unless you are accustomed to vigorous activity, you should keep your exercise heart rate below 85% MHR.

Your heart rate will act like a 'built-in' coach, telling you when to proceed in your exercise programme. As a person exercises and becomes fitter, exercise heart rate becomes lower for an equivalent workload. For example, if you start out by cycling at 15 kmph, your exercise heart rate may be 150 BPM.

However, after several weeks of regular cycling, you will discover a reduction in exercise heart rate, say to 130 BPM, while cycling at the same speed. You must then increase your cycling speed to return your heart rate to the original prescribed level.

While still a beginning exerciser, you should monitor your exercise heart rate 3 to 4 times during each session, and adjust your exercise intensity accordingly. As you become more familiar with your exercise programme, you will become familiar with your physical sensations within your training zone. Soon it will be possible for you to monitor exercise intensity just by your sense of exertion, and, thereafter, you will need to check your heart rate only occasionally.

In some sports like tennis and half-court basketball, you are almost forced to rely on your sense of exertion. The discontinuous action will cause your heart rate to go up and down—and you won't want to stop the game continually to take your pulse. If the exercise is to be beneficial in terms of general fitness, it should produce physical feelings comparable to those of an effective continuous activity, for 50-75% of the playing time. If not, you, either, need to increase play intensity (play harder or find better opponents) or consider spending more time with another sport.

DURATION: HOW MUCH TO EXERCISE

The next question you will probably ask is, 'How much do I have to do?' Articles in popular magazines, and newspaper advertisements give a variety of confusing answers. For example, one doctor claims that running a marathon (about 35 km) is the only real way a person can insure protection against heart attack; on the other hand, an advertisement for a mini-trampoline maintains that 5 minutes of bouncing each day is all the exercise anyone needs. The real answer lies somewhere in between.

Total Work or 'Calories Burned' Concept

It is impossible to prescribe one time period that will apply to all fitness exercise because duration really depends upon the intensity of action: a high intensity exercise of short duration can provide the same results as a lower intensity programme with longer duration. Put another way, when total work (calories burned) of two different activities is equal, the fitness benefits will be equal. (But there are lower limits, as we shall see in a moment.)

Dr Mike Pollock, director of the Institute for Aerobics Research, conducted a study which provides a good example of this intensity-duration relationship. For 20 weeks, two groups of men, aged 40-57, exercised and performed the same amount of total physical work. One group exercised with fast-walking (intensity 70% MHR), 40 minutes a day, 4 days per week; the other group ran (intensity 85% MHR) 30 minutes a day, 3 days per week. At the conclusion of the study, the measurable fitness benefits of the two groups were equal. This means, that, to a point, you can slow down the pace of exercise, go a little longer, and still derive the same fitness benefits. But there is a limit—the relationship is valid only when the intensity of exercise is at least 70% MHR.

Now we understand the concept of total work, but the question still remains—how much is needed? It appears that the total work completed in an exercise session should be close to 300 calories. The manner in which this is accomplished can vary: if it is continuous exercise, it can be 15-20 minutes of high intensity (90% MHR) exercise, 20-30 minutes of moderate intensity (75-85% MHR) exercise or 30-40 minutes of minimal intensity (70% MHR) exercise.

Continuous & Discontinuous Activities

If you don't enjoy continuous activities, and prefer to get your exercise from discontinuous sports, you will need longer sessions (even though there are several moments during a game when the intensity of play is maximal). The length of play will depend upon the individual sport, but the general rule of thumb would be anywhere from 40-60 minutes. (Specific duration requirements for various sports are discussed in Chapter 5).

Intensity-Duration Relationship or Time–Effective Exercises

There are a lot of arguments these days about which is the best form of exercise for general fitness. How many times have you heard a statement like, '15 minutes of jumping rope is worth 30 minutes of running'. It may or may not be true and you can easily determine the answer in a given case by checking the intensity-duration relationship. Jumping rope is, by nature, a very intense activity (90-95%

MHR) and can certainly provide the same fitness results as 30 minutes of low intensity jogging (70-75%MHR). But this does not make rope jumping a better exercise; it just makes it a more time-effective exercise. If a person ran at 90-95% MHR for 15 minutes, the fitness benefit would be exactly the same. So when you hear comparative statements, remember that there is no one best exercise. The important concept is total work performed (so long as intensity is at least 70% MHR).

Setting Optimal Duration for Exercising (How Much Exercise per Session)

Finally, a comment on the old axiom, ' if a little is good, more is better.' This is true in a theoretical sense, but it has practical limits. Probably the most important relates to the experience of many adults who have suffered muscle or bone problems when they have 'overdone it'. Sports scientists generally feel that the 300-calorie-per-session limit represents a sensible maximum. It provides good cardiovascular fitness and can be an effective amount of exercise for those seeking body fat reduction. Considering all factors, you could generalise that the optimal duration of exercise is 20-40 minutes for continuous activities and 40-60 minutes for discontinuous activities.

FREQUENCY: HOW OFTEN TO EXERCISE

Once one has answered the question of 'how much exercise per session?', there remains the question of 'how many sessions per week?' It is obvious that an afternoon of tennis will not maintain fitness for the month; but is it necessary to play every day? By experimenting with different exercise schedules, sport scientists found that the improvements in fitness are directly related to frequency of participation, but only to a point: 3-4 days per week is optimal for most adults.

During these studies, improvements were seen in cardiovascular fitness, when the subjects exercise only one or two days a week. So why the minimal recommendation of three days per week? First, to be effective, these low frequency programmes of 1-2 days per week, have to consist of very high intensity exercise (90-95%MHR) which is not suitable or enjoyable for most adults. And some who are susceptible to heart disease can actually endanger their health by exercising at this high rate or intensity. But for many people, the important point is that exercise must be pleasurable—or there just won't be a programme.

Furthermore, exercising one or two days per week seems less effective for those trying to lose body fat. Even when the total caloric expenditure was similar to a three-day-a-week programme, none of the subjects in the study lost weight.

What about the other side of the coin—exercising

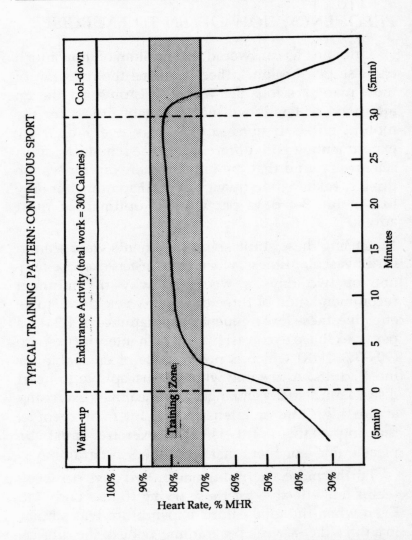

Figure 4. Heart rate response during training with a continuous sport like running, swimming, or cycling. Exercise heart rate should be between 70-85% MHR for 20-40 minutes.

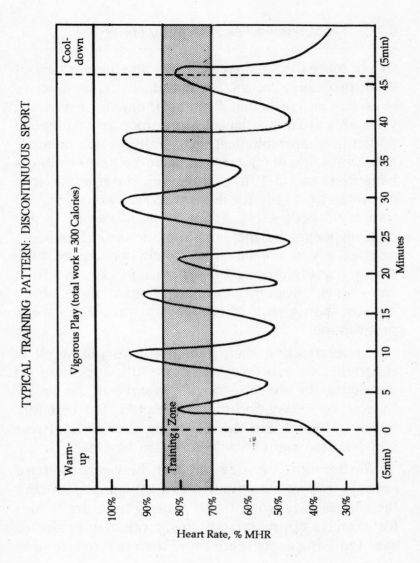

Figure 5. Heart rate response during training with a discontinuous sport like basketball, racquetball, or tennis. Exercise heart rate should exceed 70% MHR for at least 50% of playing time. Duration of play should be 40-60 minutes per session.

five or more days per week? Everyone has read about (and, probably, knows) the enthusiast who exercises everyday and feels that all is lost if one day is missed. Well, this anxiety is based more upon psychological addiction than biological fact. Training five or more times a week will not bring substantially better fitness benefits than a 3-4 times-per-week programme; it is recommended only for those who really enjoy it, and find their bodies can adapt to it. Moreover, high-frequency exercise increases the odds of orthopaedic injuries if you are not a seasoned participant. One research study reported that novice joggers in a five-day—week programme suffered three times more injuries than a similar group in a three-day—week programme.

Understanding then, that 3-4 days per week is sufficient for most of us, it is still important to distribute the exercise days throughout the week. Exercise on Friday, Saturday and Sunday will certainly improve fitness, but the following four days of rest will put you right back where you began.

Furthermore, a day of rest between exercise sessions allows the muscles to recuperate, reducing the chance of injuries. Good general rules are to aim for exercise approximately every other day, and to avoid missing exercise for more than two consecutive days.

An exception might be an exercise programme aimed at body fat reduction, where high-frequency might be worthwhile. People who are primarily concerned with losing weight, desire immediate results, and exercising 3-4 days per week offers limited caloric expenditure. The best weight loss programme often combines a moderate reduction in daily food intake (100-300 Calories) with a high-frequency exercise schedule of five or more days per week. Unfortunately, people who need to lose weight are often more prone to exercise-induced injuries; and high-frequency programmes for weight loss are, thus, often more successful when emphasising activities that are easy on the feet and knees, such as walking, swimming, or cycling, in lieu of, say—running, racquetball, or basketball. (Because of the increase in muscle mass during the beginning stages of an exercise programme, it is typical to see little weight loss for the first 4-8 weeks, even though body fat is being lost—but at least clothes will fit better.)

SUMMING UP

The two most frequently asked questions about exercise are 'What is the best kind?' and 'How much do I have to do?' To optimise health through weight control and cardiovascular fitness, the best exercise is one that involves the large leg muscles and requires stamina. Continuous sports like running, swimming and cycling are excellent; so are many discontinuous sports like tennis, racquetball and basketball, so long as they are played vigorously. (See Chapter 5 for a more complete list of effective sports.)

The proper quantity of exercise is around 300 calories per session. This will require varying amounts of time, depending upon the intensity of exercise and the continuity of action. The minimal training intensity is 70% MHR; prolonged exercise above 85% MHR increases injury risk and is not generally recommended—particularly for those who are unfit. Keeping within these intensity limits, optimal duration for continuous sports is 20-40 minutes (where intensity is 70-85% MHR), and 40-60 minutes for discontinuous sports that are played vigorously (where intensity is above 70% MHR at least 50% of the time).

Exercise quantity also implies frequency, and research supports 3-4 days per week as the optimal level. Programmes consisting of one or two days per week may result in some improved cardiovascular fitness, but will be of limited usefulness where loss of body fat is desired. Participation in excess of 5 days per week is possible for those who are fit, but will increase the chance of injury for the novice. High-frequency programmes are useful for people serious about weight loss, but non-jarring exercises like walking, swimming, or cycling are recommended to avoid leg injuries.

3

Look Before You Leap:
How Safe Is It To Exercise

IT IS DANGEROUS NOT TO EXERCISE

People can, at times, be very spontaneous. Frequently, they try to erase years of inactivity with one Sunday morning tennis game or one Saturday morning run. For most of these enthusiasts, muscle aches and joint pains will be the price for doing too much too soon. For a few, it may mean serious danger to their hearts.

Because the rare jogging heart attacks always get a 'good press', many would-be sports participants question, logically, the safety of exercise. To them, it seems reasonable that exercise is dangerous: it forces the heart to beat fast and work hard. And their friends who run or bicycle regularly are always talking about that 'cardiac hill'.

Exercise can be dangerous for certain people, but only for a few. The American Heart Association predicts that 10 per cent of males over age 35 have a hidden heart disease. Even for most of these, proper exercise is not harmful; in some cases, it may even reduce heart abnormalities.

Taking everything into account and remembering the points discussed in Chapter 1, we can conclude that, for most people, it is more dangerous *not* to exercise.

WHEN IS A PRE-EXERCISE MEDICAL CHECK-UP NECESSARY?

It is generally recommended, that you visit a doctor before undertaking a serious exercise programme. This is not a blanket rule—medical evaluation is more important for some than others. If you are under the age of 30, have constantly remained in good health and have been exercising two to three times per week for years, the medical evaluation would represent an abundance of caution. But for those over 30, the chances of heart disease begin to rise, and for anyone who has not been recently examined, a pre-exercise check-up becomes a must. In fact, for those over 30— if you are in perfect health and exercising regularly— it is wise to repeat a physical examination once every other year.

PRE-EXERCISE MEDICAL QUESTIONNAIRE

If You Answer 'Yes' To Any Question— Consult Your Doctor.

1. Has your doctor ever said you have heart trouble?

2. Do you frequently have pains in your chest?

3. Have you ever had an abnormal electrocardiogram (ECG), either, while resting or exercising?

4. Have you ever had sensations of irregular or 'skipped' heart beats?

5. Do you often feel faint or have severe dizziness?

6. Do you have diabetes, high cholesterol, a family history of heart disease or do you smoke more than a pack and a half of cigarettes a day?

7. Has a doctor ever said your blood pressure is too high?

8. Has a doctor ever told you that you have a bone or joint problem that has been aggravated by exercise?

9. Are you over the age of 60 and not accustomed to vigorous exercise?

10. Is there any other physical reason which you know of, due to which, you should not, perhaps, get into an active physical programme even if you want to?

Telling you to visit a doctor and having you actually go are two different matters. Paying for a medical evaluation when one is completely healthy, goes against anyone's grain. It is an unfortunate fact, but most people never think or do anything about their health until they lose it. So, for those who are contemplating 'hedging their bets', I have included a special medical history Questionnaire. If you answer 'yes' to any of these questions, no matter what be your age, it is mandatory that you visit a doctor before engaging in vigorous exercise.

The Medical Evaluation: Your Personal Risk Assessment Score

Be sure your doctor understands the purpose of the medical evaluation ahead of time. Remember, the point is to find out if there is any good medical reason why you should limit your participation in regular vigorous exercise. The strategy behind a medical evaluation designed for 'exercise clearance' is different from that used in a routine examination designed to check general health. For instance, the physician will probably want to know more about your past history of exercise, and whether you have ever had bone, muscle or joint problems. The examination should also include various questions and tests that will estimate the current risk of coronary heart disease.

Age, sex, and family history of heart disease are

all possible risk factors, as are certain biological characteristics and personal habits. *Figure 6* outlines these variables in detail, and allows one to compile a total risk score. Your physician will probably perform this analysis without the use of a chart, but be assured these are the variables he or she is thinking about. Also remember, only a doctor is qualified to interpret the results and decide whether or not it is safe for you to start an exercise programme.

ECG and Treadmill Tests

One test that should be a part of every pre-exercise medical evaluation is the electrocardiogram (ECG). The ECG provides valuable information about the condition of the heart by recording small electrical impulses that are normally transmitted with each beat. A heart can sound and feel very normal to a doctor, while the ECG may discover a defect he can't hear, such as a significant clogging in the coronary arteries. Obviously, this would be important knowledge to have before beginning an exercise programme.

The ECG can be performed, either, while you are lying down or while you are exercising (stress ECG). The resting ECG comes first. It will uncover any obvious abnormality, thereby, making it unwise to have the exercise ECG first. For most people the resting ECG will turn out normal; but it will only have monitored the heart at rest and will not provide

HEART DISEASE RISK FACTOR ANALYSIS

RISK FACTORS	SCORE 0	1	2	3	4	5	6	Your Score
Systolic[1] Blood pressure (mm Hg)	110 or less	120	130	140	150	160	170 or more	
Diastolic[2] Blood Pressure (mm Hg)	70 or less	80	85	90	95	100	105 or more	
Cigarettes/ day	None past 4 years	None past 1 year	5	10	20	30	40 or more	
Cholesterol (mg%)	180 or less	200	220	230	250	275	290 or more	
Triglycerides (mg%)	80 or less	100	120	150	200	250	300 or more	
Age and Sex	Female under 40	Male under 40	Female 40-55	Female over 55	Male 40-50	Male 50-60	Male over 60	
Heredity (Blood relatives under age 60)	0		1	2	3	4	5 or more	

	Lean	Normal	Slightly Over-weight	Very Over-weight		
Weight						
Vigorous Exercise (Days/Week)	4 or more	3	2	1	0	
Stress-Tension	Almost Never	Occasional	Frequent	Almost Constant		
Diabetes	No					Yes

Your Total Score = ___

Your Total Score	Your Risk Assessment
If your score is 0-5	A very low risk of heart disease
" 6-16	Low risk
" 17-25	Moderate risk
" 26-34	High risk
" 35+	Very high risk

Figure 6.

1. Blood pressure during a heart contraction when blood is pumped into the arteries.
2. Blood pressure during the period between 2 contractions of the heart when the heart relaxes and allows the chambers to fill with blood.

important information about the heart when it is put under the stress of exercise.

For all people over the age of 30, it is highly recommended that an exercise ECG be completed in addition to the resting ECG. As the name implies, it monitors heart action while you are exercising— usually, while you step up and down on a bench, ride a bicycle or walk on a motor-driven treadmill. The stress test checks out the body's response to such exercise; it may turn up problems at high heart rates, which would raise serious questions about further exercise or make it advisable to reduce or limit the exercise programme.

Not all doctors are equipped to perform an exercise stress test. If yours isn't, have him do your resting ECG, and then ask for a referral. Many hospitals and medical colleges now provide exercise stress tests to the general public at very reasonable fees.

Once all the test results are in, the doctor can evaluate your readiness for an exercise programme. Sometimes exercise is not recommended at all, but this happens quite rarely. Sometimes, the prescription will be for temporary or limited restrictions on exercise. For example, a person with very high blood pressure should not exercise until the level is reduced, by medication and/or weight loss. The doctor will permit exercise when he feels that blood pressure is under control, though he may suggest starting with a professionally supervised programme. Organised programmes can be found at many YMCAs, colleges, and hospitals. In most cases, however, the doctor will report a good medical evaluation and be glad to recommend exercise.

Unfortunately, most physicians are extremely busy with unhealthy patients, and do not have the time to explain all the details involved in a good programme. They are very concerned, however, that you 'use common sense' and 'do not overdo it'. While these are good general guidelines, the beginner needs more information.

That's what this book is for—between your doctor's advice and the information contained in the following chapters, you have everything you need.

LISTEN TO YOUR BODY: RECOGNIZING THE DANGER SIGNALS

After you start an exercise programme or even if you have been exercising regularly for years, it is important to be aware of body symptoms that could indicate something is wrong. Usually your only problems are common aches and pains in your muscles and joints. These symptoms indicate that you are doing too much and need to reduce your level of exercise. But some symptoms are associated with very serious problems; if you experience any of them, *stop exercising and consult a physician before resuming*. These symptoms include:

Abnormal heart action : Be aware of your heart beat; it should be very regular. Watch for fluttering, jumping or sudden pounding sensations in the chest or throat. Sometimes heart irregularities result in a sensation of sudden loss of breath (lasting one or two seconds). You should check your heart every now and then, feeling your pulse, either, on your chest wall or at your wrist. Watch for sudden increases or decreases in heart rate.

Listen to Your Body's Warning Signals

If you experience any of the following symptoms, you are overexerting, and should reduce your amount of exercise.

1. Extreme breathlessness 5 to 10 minutes, after finishing exercise.
2. Prolonged fatigue or loss of energy.
3. Insomnia.
4. Nausea immediately after exercise.
5. Prolonged rapid heart rate (110 beats per minutes or greater) 5 to 10 minutes after exercise.
6. Persistent muscle or joint pain (may not occur until the following day).

Chest pains: Sensation of tightness, pressure, squeezing pain, or heaviness are serious body symptoms, especially when they are caused by exercise and only disappear gradually with rest (5-15 minutes). The chest cavity is the main area to watch, but similar pain in the throat, jaw, or left arm can indicate the same serious problem. Note: chest pain is not always felt during exercise; it may occur anytime. It is always a reason for concern.

Dizziness: This symptom indicates insufficient blood flow to the brain, and is especially serious during exercise. Other similar sensations include lightheadedness, sudden loss of coordination, confusion or fainting. If you experience one of these symptoms, immediately lie down and elevate your feet. Note: sometimes dizziness is experienced right after vigorous exercise. This is somewhat common and does not usually indicate a serious problem. To avoid post-exercise dizzines, stay active for 5 to 10 minutes after your workout—say, by walking briskly—before you sit down or shower. If the problem persists, see your doctor.

Anyone can experience a variety of body symptoms which are not associated with serious medical problems, but are your body's way of telling you to slow down. In these cases, try to remedy the situation alone before seeking a physician's advice. It's natural to want to be a hero, especially when 'running around' outdoors, but you can not fool your body—listen to it.

SUMMING UP

For most people, proper exercise presents no danger to health. To minimise risk, however, it is recommended that all persons over 30, consult a physician before attempting vigorous exercise. Inform the doctor of your intentions, so he can focus on those tests and questions that relate to coronary heart disease. Remember, only a physician is qualified to interpret risk of heart disease and to decide whether or not exercise is safe for you. When you exercise, always be sensitive to any physical symptoms that could indicate health problems, particularly any abnormal heart action, chest pain or dizziness. When these occur, stop exercising immediately and consult a physician.

4
Getting Started

Modern technology, with its multitude of work-saving devices, has virtually eliminated the need for human muscle power. Physical activity used to be necessary for life and survival, but is now thought of only as recreation, and has to, therefore, compete with other leisure time activities. Unfortunately, people have adapted well to this sedentary existence, and often avoid exercise because it seems too hard or inconvenient. Those who do stretch their muscles on occasion are quickly discouraged when the next morning's aches and pains remind them of years of inactivity.

These negative experiences are common when starting out, and make the establishment of an exercise programme difficult. But the human body can adapt to habitual exercise, just as it has adapted to sedentary living. The key to success is approaching it gradually—a slow exposure to increasing amounts of exercise. Often, people who have never exercised in their life become 'addicted', to the point where they become physically and mentally upset if a scheduled exercise session is missed. At this point, it's the other daily obligations that become inconvenient, disrupting scheduled tennis matches or swimming workouts.

Ideally, almost everyone could become addicted to exercise. To a large extent, it just takes 'getting into it'. Depending on the individual, it can take anywhere from 2 to 4 months before regular exercise feels comfortable and part of the normal routine.

The first month of this adaptation period is particularly difficult and requires a special plan of attack. 'Getting started' is what this chapter is all about. The following sections discuss various techniques, both physical and mental, that will help smooth the road to success. Read them carefully and apply them patiently.

Making It Convenient: Adapting Exercise to Suit Your Lifestyle

Exercise will soon be abandoned unless it is relatively convenient. Obviously the best solution is to make physical activity a necessary part of the day—like using a bicycle for transportation instead of a car. But this is not always practical, so other forms of exercise must be found that can easily fit into the normal routine. However, there are many factors to consider—time of day, season, availability of shower facilities, and location of exercise area—all affect the convenience of exercise. Since everyone faces a different set of circumstances, no one solution is suggested. Your final decision must be based on your personality and lifestyle.

Convenience is rarely a problem on the weekend, but during the week the demands of one's occupation and other obligations can present tough obstacles. Many people exercise before breakfast because there are never any interruptions and a shower is generally available. For those who are not 'morning people', exercise during the noon hour or after work are the next logical choices. The important point is to discover your most convenient time, and then faithfully adhere to your schedule, so exercise will become a routine habit.

The type of sport or exercise you select also has an effect on programme convenience. Individual sports like running and cycling are obviously more convenient than team sports like soccer and basketball. Many times, a favourite sport is not the most convenient one. Bad weather can eliminate favourite activities. When in need, select one or two other sports from Chapter 5-6 to supplement your 'convenient' sport when conditions require an alternative. This will help ensure regular exercise.

Avoid Too Much Too Soon

Generally when a person begins an exercise programme, his lungs can accommodate the stress much better than his muscles or joints. Therefore, an exercise that feels comfortable may actually be damaging connective tissues in the legs; and the damage may not cause pain until the next day or next week. Such orthopaedic injuries constitute the number-one reason why people drop out of exercise programmes, and they must be avoided! The cause is, simply—doing too much too soon. The solution is to start slowly and progress gradually—much more gradually than you would like to.

Exercise Starter Programme

If you have never exercised on a regular basis or if you are over 30 and have been inactive for the past 6 months, a special 5-week Starter Programme is mandatory for injury prevention (see *Figure 7*). Such a programme involves a combination of walking and jogging, and is important for two reasons: first, walking and jogging are convenient forms of exercise that can be performed mostly anywhere, anytime, with or without a partner. Second, this type of muscular action stresses the feet, ankles and knees, and is the best exercise (when done properly) to prepare the legs for more extensive running or other vigorous sports.

5-WEEK WALK JOG STARTER PROGRAMME

This 5 week Walk-Jog Starter Programme has been designed to strengthen lower body musculature—for those unaccustomed to vigorous exercise.

FW	SJ	FW	SJ	FW	SJ	FW	SJ	FW	SJ	FW	SJ	FW	SJ	Total Time Spent (in minutes)
1st Week (Do only once)														
20 min														20
2nd Week (Do Thrice, preferably alternate days)														
2 min	0.5 min	2	0.5	2	0.5	2	0.5	2	0.5	2	0.5	2	0.5	20
3rd Week (Six Times)														
2 min	1 min	2	1	2	1	2	1	2	1					18
4th Week (Four Times)														
2 min	2 min	2	2	2	2	2	2							16
5th Week (Five Times)														
1 min	2 min	1	2	1	2	1	2	1	2					15

Figure 7

FW = Fast Walk
SJ = Slow Jog

You will quickly discover that the Starter Programme may not require sufficient exercise intensity to elevate heart rate to the training zone of 70-85%MHR. In this respect, it does not satisfy the principles outlined in Chapter 2. However, the primary objective of the Starter Programme is to strengthen the leg muscles, and this must take precedence during the initial period. After 5 weeks, you may progress to your favourite sport (consult Chapter 5), gradually building up intensity, duration, and frequency according to the principles set out in Chapter 2.

If you have been exercising on a regular basis, the Starter Programme is not required. Be very sensitive, however, to any signs of leg injuries. If they do occur, stop exercising for a week (or switch to an activity that puts no strain on the injury), and then resume your original programme. If the pain reappears, stop (or switch) again for a week, but this time, begin with the Starter Programme (because your legs need more strength).

Swimming and cycling have their own special Starter Programme. Neither of these sports puts stress on the legs like running or jumping, so they do not require the Walk-Jog Starter Programme. If you plan to concentrate on these sports, go directly to the sport programmes outlined in Chapter 5-6. As indicated, swimming and cycling are good substitute sports for people recovering from injuries sustained in other activities.

Committing Yourself

The most difficult part of an exercise programme is not the physical activity, but learning how to adhere to 3-4 day/week regimen. For weekend athletes, the addition of one or two exercise days during the week is only a minor challenge. However, those of you who have only been 'getting out' once or twice a year face a major change in lifestyle.

The only way to begin is to jump in and start (right foot in front of left and so on...). But there are a few tricks that might help you hang on during the crucial early adjustment period.

First, make a serious commitment to regular exercise for 5 weeks. Choose the starting date wisely: a time when you will not be travelling or running into other conflicts. Jumping into an exercise programme on a whim does not allow appropriate time to prepare mentally, and excuses for missing sessions come too easily.

When you design your 5-week plan, you may want to write it down in detail, including the exact days and times for exercise. For some this may be too restrictive, and more irritating than helpful. The important point is to carefully map out a plan, and then stick to it.

The successful completion of your 5-week exercise commitment plays a vital part in helping you develop a permanent exercise programme. Therefore, a few suggestions are offered on how to strengthen this important commitment:

Exercise Motivation Boosters

1. Make your plans known to your spouse or a close friend and solicit his/her encouragement.

2. Set up immediate rewards, like a favourite activity, for completing each scheduled exercise.

3. Think about how your health and fitness is improving with each exercise session.

4. If you can afford it, buy attractive exercise clothes and equipment. They can help you feel like a champion athlete, and may also inspire you to exercise to get some use out of your investment in them.

5. Put more sport into your life: buy a subscription to a popular sport magazine; see more professional games; talk with your friends about sports and your exercise programme.

Putting it all together: Warming Up, Cardio-vascular & Cooling Down Exercises

There is an old saying: 'If you are going to take the time to do something, do it right.' Well, an exercise programme is just not 'right' unless each session includes three basic components (see *Figures 4* and *5*, Chapter 2):

		Time (min.)
1.	Warm-up	5
2.	Cardiovascular exercise	20-60
3.	Cool-down	5

The cardiovascular exercise is still the heart of your programme, and, therefore, absolutely necessary. The other two components, the warm-up and cool-down, require a few extra minutes, but they make the difference between a good exercise programme and an excellent one. To ignore them is like buying a ten-thousand-dollar car without a radio, to save two-hundred dollars.

Warming Up

The warm-up routine consists of ten floor exercises, nine flexibility exercises and one abdominal strength exercise (pages 63-75). These five minutes of passive stretching prepare the body for vigorous activity by loosening muscles and lubricating joints. Many minor aches and pains are created when a cold or stiff muscle is forced to exercise; a proper warm-up can definitely reduce the risk of injures.

Also, the cardiovascular system responds better to exercise after a warm-up period. Research has shown that sudden exposure to high-intensity exercise can cause heart irregularities in normal, healthy people. When the same individuals exercised after several minutes of warm-up activity, there were significantly fewer heart irregularities. (Most people, probably, are not in any real danger if they plunge right into sudden heavy exercise, but it makes sense to be prudent. And, in addition, many people find it easier to get into exercise gradually, without the strain of starting out cold.)

Low back pain, a common problem for thousands of people, can often be remedied or avoided with a conscientious and well-selected warm-up routine. Poor posture, inflexible back and leg muscles, and weak abdominal muscles all contribute to misaligned vertebrae and eventual chronic back pain. The Forward Bend and Lower Back Stretch exercises (see pp. 69, 72) lengthen back muscles that are attached to the vertebrae, and can relieve the pulling pressure that causes pinched nerves. A protruding stomach can also put stress on the backbone and pinch nerves, and Bent Knee Sit-ups (see p. 73) will strengthen abdominal muscles and provide relief. Note: if the warm-up exercises cause or increase back pain, stop all activity, and consult your physician before resuming.

The warm-up routine should be completed just prior to your cardiovascular exercise period. Use the full five minutes and perform the exercises in the order they are listed.

The best method for stretching is to slowly bend until you first feel the muscle pull; then stop and hold that position for 3-5 seconds. Bouncing or jerking motions can injure tissues and cause residual pain—do not, therefore, bounce!

After completing the warm-up routine, it is still wise to work slowly into the cardiovascular exercise. Think of the first 1-3 minutes as an extension of the warm-up period. For tennis players, this means slow easy rallies at first, before all out play. For runners and swimmers, this means a gradual build-up to training speed.

The human body is a durable item, but it must be treated with care and respect.

WARM-UP EXERCISES

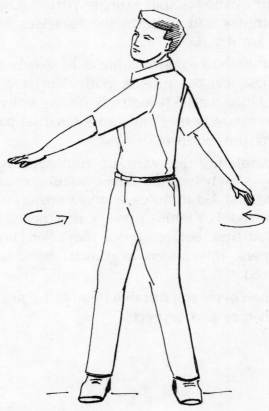

1. TRUNK TWISTER

Starting Position: Stand with feet pointing forward, shoulder-width apart, arms extended.

Action: Twist upper body to the right as far as possible, and then immediately twist to the left (do not hold twisted position). Avoid lifting heels.

Time: Continue twisting right and left for 30 seconds.

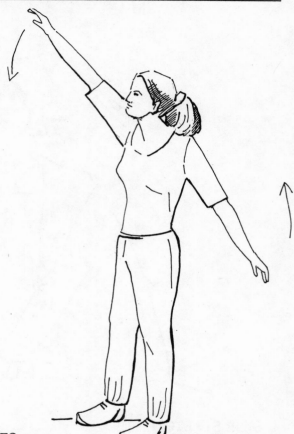

2. ARM CIRCLES

Starting position: Stand with feet pointing forward, shoulder-width apart, one arm extended straight up and the other straight down.

Action: Rotate both arms forward in maximum circles. Then reverse, and rotate arms in a backward direction. (Keep arms straight.)

Time: Rotate in each direction for 15 seconds.

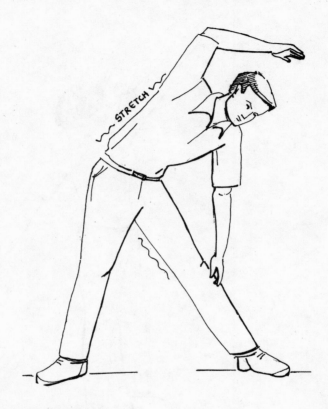

STRETCH

3. SIDE STRETCH

Starting position: Stand erect with right arm raised (with
elbow bent) and left arm by the side,
feet pointing forward, somewhat more
than the shoulder-width apart.

Action: Bend upper body to the left until
muscles first pull; hold position for a
few seconds. Return to starting
position and repeat to the right.

Time: Alternate bending right and left for 30
seconds.

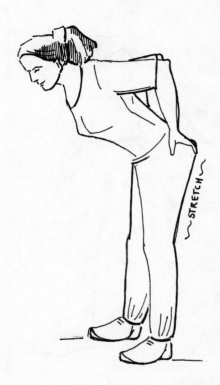

STRETCH

4. FORWARD BEND

Starting position: Stand with hands on hips, feet pointing forward, shoulder-width apart.

Action: Keeping back straight, slowly bend forward at the waist until muscle tension is first noticed; hold position for a few seconds. Return to starting position and repeat.

Time: Repeat for 30 seconds.

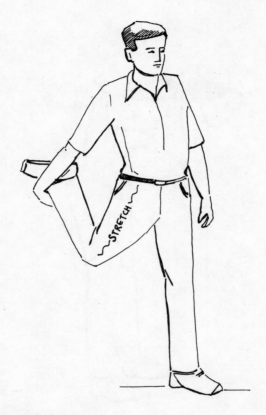

5. THIGH STRETCH

Starting position: Stand with feet pointing forward, shoulder-width apart.

Action: Lift right foot and grasp right ankle with right hand. Pull right heel back and upward toward buttocks until muscle tension is first noticed; hold position for a few seconds.

Time: Alternate stretching right and left thighs for 30 seconds.

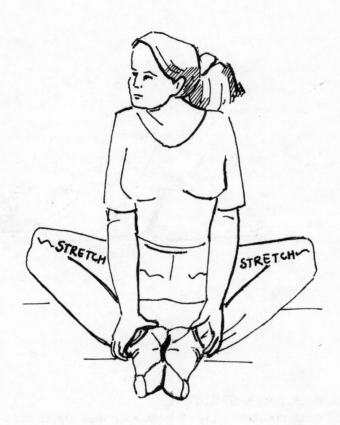

6. GROIN STRETCH

Starting position: Sit with knees pointing outward and bottom of feet placed together.

Action: Grasp ankles and lean forward until muscle tension is first noticed; hold position for a few seconds. Return to starting position and repeat.

Time: Repeat for 30 seconds.

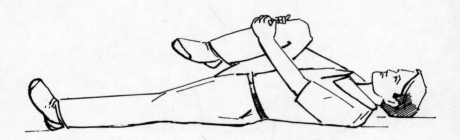

7.   LOWER BACK STRETCH

Starting position :   Lie on back with legs together.

Action :   Lift right knee and pull it with both hands towards the chest until muscle tension is first noticed; hold position for a few seconds. Return to starting position and repeat with left knee.

Time :   Alternate pulling right and left leg for 30 seconds.

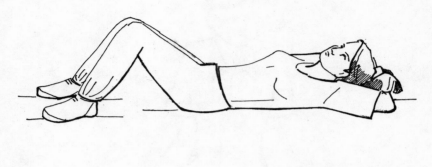

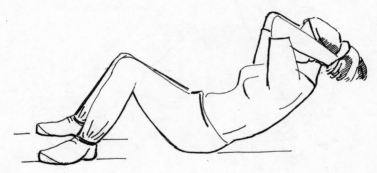

8. BENT KNEE SIT-UP

Starting position: Lie on back with hands behind head; knees bent with feet flat on ground, shoulder-width apart.

Action: Sit-up slightly (45 degrees) until stomach muscles tighten; hold position for a few seconds. Return to starting position and repeat.

Time: Repeat for 30 seconds.

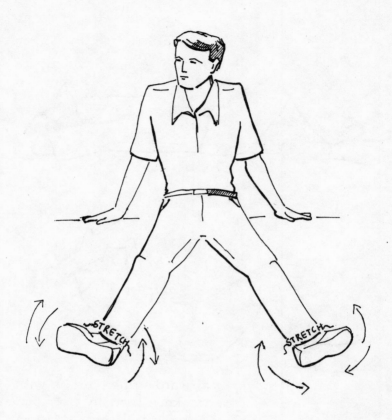

9. FEET CIRCLES

Starting position: Sit with legs extended and feet more than shoulder-width apart; hands on group behind for support.

Action: Keeping heels on ground, rotate both feet at the same time in maximum circles. Rotate feet in opposite direction.

Time : Each direction for 15 seconds.

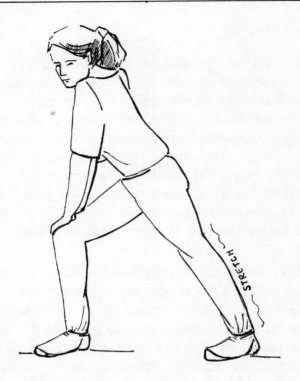

10. CALF STRETCH

Starting position: Stand in forward stride position with the forward knee partially bent and the rear knee locked straight; feet pointed forward separated by more than shoulder width; heels flat on the ground.

Action: Lean forward until muscle tension is first noticed; hold position for a few seconds. Return to starting position and repeat with other leg forward.

Time: Alternate stretching right and left calf for 30 seconds.

Cooling Down

A five-minute period of gradual recovery after vigorous exercise is just as important as the pre-exercise warm-up. During this time you should walk briskly or jog lightly, so that your heart rate, breathing and body temperature can gradually return to normal resting levels. For those plagued with muscle tightness, it is a good ideal also to repeat the warm-up exercises. (This technique of stretching, both, before and after exercise, has proved helpful in reducing muscle soreness, and is now used by major track teams.)

Sudden cessation of vigorous exercise may cause blood to accumulate in the enlarged vessels of the legs. (Vessels swell during exercise to dissipate heat.) Without muscular contractions to squeeze this blood upward, blood flow to the heart and brain will slow down, and may result in dizziness, feeling faint, and irregular heart beats. The light activity of a cool-down period will maintain proper circulation until the leg blood vessels contract to normal size, and avoid these symptoms (known as 'blood pooling').

The heat from a hot shower, sauna, steam bath, or whirlpool can also enlarge blood vessels and lead to blood pooling, so it makes sense to avoid them right after vigorous exercise. (If you are hurried for time, a luke warm or cool shower is the best solution.) Exposure to hot water or steam from these various facilities may be hazardous for some people even after they have fully recovered from exercise. Therefore, when using this 'health' equipment, be sensitive to any signs of lightheadedness, dizziness or irregular heart beats. Never use a steam room or sauna alone; always bring a friend.

Poor circulation is also a primary cause of residual muscle pain. Blood-born lactic acid, a normal metabolic by-product of exercise, will cause muscle soreness unless it is quickly removed. Light muscular activity enhances circulation, and ensures that lactic acid is carried away.

Finally, the cool-down period offers a unique reward for a job well done. The acute sensation of relaxation has been likened to an alcoholic 'buzz', except that the physical senses are sharpened instead of dulled. This is a time when optimism pervades and life really feels good. Relax and contemplate these positive sensations. Exercise is a rare experience—it not only feels good, it is actually good for you.

SUMMING UP

The hardest part of an exercise programme is not the physical activity, but learning how to adhere to a 3-4 day—week regimen. When starting out, the first one-two months are critical, while you shape future exercise habits and attitudes. A well-thought-out plan of attack is very important—one where convenience is the primary concern. For people unaccustomed to vigorous activity, a special 5-week Starter Programme is effective. Make a strong personal commitment to your plan and stay with it.

A complete exercise programme includes three basic components: warm-up (5 min.), cardiovascular exercise (20-60 min.) and cool-down (5 min.). The cardiovascular exercise is necessary for heart health and, often, for weight control. The warm-up and cool-down periods are designed to increase the safety and comfort of vigorous exercise, while reducing orthopaedic injuries and muscle soreness. The human body is a durable item, but it must be treated with care and respect.

5

Exercises For Cardiovascular Fitness: The Continuous Sports

There is no one magical sport. Cardiovascular fitness and weight control benefits can be achieved through a great variety of activities. The important qualifications of a good fitness sport were outlined in Chapter 2:

1. Primarily using large leg muscles;
2. Continuous action for at least 50-75% of the exercise time;
3. Expenditure of approximately 300 Calories in 20-60 minutes;
4. Intensity level at 70-85% MHR.

This chapter lists the many sports that meet these

fitness qualifications. Popular activities will be discussed in some details; less popular but effective fitness sports are listed in the Fitness Activities Chart in the following chapter. With the popular sport, references are cited which will provide additional information on specific sport skills, strategy, warm-up, and muscular strength exercises. The more you learn about a sport, the greater the enjoyment.

A good exercise programme may revolve around just one sport or it may include two or three sports used on different days or different times of the year. Some people even enjoy mixing sports during each session: for example, jumping properly for 10 minutes, then running for 10 minutes, followed by 10 minutes of swimming. The combination doesn't matter, so long as approximately 300 Calories are burned at the intensity of 70-85% MHR. The exercise programme that you decide upon will take one of these forms, depending upon your personal interest and the activity's convenience. The important point, once again, is to develop a regular exercise habit, of sessions 3-4 times a week.

A continuous sport is one that demands steady, continual muscular action. Running, cycling and swimming are prime examples. These types of sports are very time efficient; that is, expending 300 Calories may take only 20-30 minutes, whereas, as we discussed earlier, discontinuous sports generally require 40-60 minutes. The greatest advantage of continuous sports is the control of exercise intensity. You can slow down your running pace, but you can't control a discontinuous sport like basketball. With personal control over intensity, you can work on your fitness at a pace that is comfortable, and without undue risk of orthopaedic injury.

Fitness Progression Levels

The following discussion on specific continuous sports contains special Fitness Progression Programmes. For each sport, there are eight exercise levels. The goal is to advance all the way to the fitness maintenance level—the lower levels will not maintain fitness and, are instead, designed to provide a comfortable and safe progression to the final permanent programme.

The speed of progression through the eight levels depends primarily on age. Research has shown that adaptation to exercise takes approximately 40 per cent longer for each decade of life after age 30. Therefore, in general, those under 30 can progress after every 4 exercise days, whereas those aged 30, 40 and 50 must progress more slowly, with 6, 8 and 11 exercise days at each progression level.

It is important to note that these age-adjusted progression rates represent minimal requirements— some need to remain longer at one or more exercise levels before moving on. When you do move on, you must confirm your readiness to do so by applying two tests on the first day at the new exercise level:

1. Your exercise heart rate must not exceed 90% MHR; and

2. The exercise session must not feel excessively difficult or leave you worn out for the rest of the day.

If you fail one of these tests, drop back a level for another week before trying to move up again. Do not be discouraged if you appear to be trapped at a particular level. Plateaus are common, but progress will come if you are patient. Remember, the important part is not the speed of progression, but sticking to the 3-4 days of exercise per week.

Your starting exercise level depends upon your exercise history. People who have been inactive for 6 months or more, and are beginning a running programme, should first complete the Walk-Jog Starter Programme outlined in Chapter 4 and then begin at Level I in the Progression Programme. Cycling (road and stationary) and swimming are different; since they differ from running, they have specific starting programmes (p. 85 and p. 91). If you have no interest in running, but enjoy walking, omit the Walk-Jog Starter Programme and start with Level 1 of the Walking Programme (p. 94)

An exercise programme utilising two, three or even four different sports is acceptable, but progression advances in one sport do not mean you are ready for automatic progression in another sport. While there is some cross-over conditioning between sports, generally, the muscles involved are different, and sport progression must be based on specific sport participation. For example, if a runner who normally does 5 km 4 times a week, wanted to add swimming to his exercise programme, he would start at swimming Level I.

Cycling: Stationary and Road

Caloric expenditure during cycling depends more on mechanical gears and the terrain, than on actual distance travelled. Therefore, instead of outlining specific distances and time (as in the Running Fitness Progression), the Cycling Programme simply requires that you keep exercise heart rate in the training zone (70-85% MHR) for specific amounts of time.

On a stationary bicycle, evaluate your exercise heart rate while pedalling. Road cycling involves more skill and balance; so it is necessary to stop completely for the heart rate check. By the time you reach the Maintenance Level, your sensations of exertion will give you a reliable measure of your exercise intensity.

If you haven't been on a bicycle for some time, start with the Cycling Starter Programme. Your thigh muscles perform most of the work in cycling, and a long gradual conditioning is necessary to avoid pain and injury. But once you become conditioned to cycling, the localised muscular action provides excellent leg strength, and will complement other sports like basketball, skiing, and tennis.

Most athletic and health clubs have stationary bicycles. For the real enthusiast, home models can be purchased from major department stores for Rs. 2,500-5,000. Be sure the stationary bike you use is well-built and has a knob or lever that can increase wheel resistance. Changing wheel resistance is the main way to control exercise intensity. Cycling faster will also increase intensity, but as you become more fit, the sufficiently high pedal speeds necessary at low resistance levels, are hard to maintain.

Stationary cycling can be very convenient, and a perfect exercise for rainy days. On the other hand, the monotony of cycling in an open place can make it very boring. You can conquer this problem by combining other diverting activities with your cycling. Try talking to a friend; some people watch television; others catch up on their reading.

The Cycling Fitness Progression will be easy to follow if you live in a flat, rural area. Hills and cross streets can make this, otherwise, continuous sport quite discontinuous. The point is to try and keep the cycling pace continuous and consistent. If there are breaks, only count the time spent cycling above 70% MHR. Sometimes it will take a 30-40 minute ride to achieve 20 minutes of real exercise. Remember, coasting down-hill is fun, but does not improve cardiovascular fitness or burn extra calories.

5-WEEK CYCLING STARTER PROGRAMME
Road or Stationary

	Cycling Days per Week	Cycling Time (min.) per session	Intensity (%MHR)	Rest Time (min.) between Cycling sessions	Repeat Cycling sessions	Total Cycling + Rest Time (min.)
1st Week	3	2	70%	2	Twice	6
2nd Week	3	3	70%	3	Twice	9
3rd Week	4	4	70%	3	Twice	11
4th Week	4	5	70%	2	Twice	12
5th Week	4	6	70%	1	Twice	13

CYCLING PROGRESSION PROGRAMME
(Road or Stationary)

Level	Intensity (%MHR)	Total Time, Each Session (min.)
I	70-85%	13
II	70-85%	14
III	70-85%	15
IV	70-85%	16
V	70-85%	17
VI	70-85%	18
VII	70-85%	19
VIII	70-85%	20
Maintenance	70-85%	20-30

MINIMUM PROGRESSION*
(Exercise 3-4 days a week)

Age	Exercise Days At Each Level	Caloric Cost	
		Weight kg	Calories per min. at 20 kmph
Below 30	4	57	9.0
30-39	6	68	10.9
40-49	8	80	12.7
50 and above	11	90	14.6

* Remember to check your readiness for each new exercise level. See p. 81-82.

Running

The constant 'pounding' action of this sport is stressful to the feet, legs and back, so a gradual introduction is important. That's why the Walk-Jog Starter Programme recommends slow jogging for short periods of time. (By definition, a jog utilises running action, but propels the body at walking speed 6-8 km per hour.) Running speeds of 10 and 11 kmph should be avoided until the Fitness Progression.

Running is a sport, where doing too much too soon, will cause injury and keep you from becoming a real runner. It is common to feel energetic at the start of a run and to want to burst into high gear. Likewise, many people want to sprint home to the barn at the end of a run, with the feeling that they are, somehow, doing something extra towards achieving a high level of fitness. Both actions are foolish; they offer few physical benefits and can be very debilitating to the bones and muscles. A good motto for the runner is 'start slow and taper off at the end.'

Good running shoes are a must, no matter what the price. Tennis shoes or cheap sneakers are the surest way to ruin a running career. Buy your running shoes at a sports shop or athletic shoes store. There are many good brands; select the one that feels most comfortable.

Finally, running is an excellent sport for the heart, but it has a negative effect on flexibility. Leg and back muscles become tight, and if left unattended to,

RUNNING

Level	Fast Walk Time (min)	Run Distance (in kms)	Run Time (min.)	Repetitions	Total Time (min.)
I	4	0.8	6	2	20
II	6	1.6	11	1	17
III	7	1.6	10	1	17
IV	5	2.4	15	1	20
V	5	2.4	14	1	19
VI	1	3.2	19	1	20
VII	1	3.2	18	1	19
VIII		4.0	22	1	22
Maintenance		4-6.4	20-35	1	20-35

MINIMUM PROGRESSION*
(Exercise 3-4 days a week)

Age	Exercise Days At Each Level	Weight kg	Caloric Cost Calories per min. at 11.0 kmph	Caloric Cost Calories per min. at 13.0 kmph
Below 30	4	57	10.6	12.1
30-39	6	68	12.7	14.5
40-49	8	80	14.8	16.9
50 and above	11	90	16.9	19.3

---

* Remember to check your readiness for each new exercise level. See p. 81-82.

can pull the hip and vertebra out of alignment. Moreover, running the next day with stiff muscles is the perfect way to injure them and disable yourself. So be sure to do the Warm-up Routine faithfully before each run. Spend a little extra time stretching the lower back and legs. You can get additional relief from muscle tightness by repeating the Warm-up Routine after each run and on non-running days.

Swimming

Swimming is a unique sport that has advantages and disadvantages compared to running. On the plus side, swimming provides optimal cardiovascular and weight control benefits without risk of leg injury. Many people who feel awkward and uncomfortable while running find this non-weight-bearing sport delightfully easy. For this same reason, swimming is the perfect substitute activity for otherwise land-bound athletes recovering from hip, knee and ankle problems.

But, whereas, swimming does wonders for upper body strength, it is not so good for the lower-body (anti-gravity) musculature of the body. Obviously, swimmers don't fall down when they climb out of the pool, but their performance in land sports is definitely compromised by a total swimming programme. On the other hand, a combination of swimming and running makes an excellent programme for all around muscular development.

Breaststroke, backstroke, butterfly, and freestyle are the acceptable swimming strokes for the Progression Programme. Sidestroke and other floating strokes are less vigorous, and not useful for general conditioning. A proper swimming technique is a must for fitness development as well as sport enjoyment. The Caloric Cost of the Swimming chart (p. 92) assumes average or good skill level. If you need basic instructions, many fine adult swimming courses are available at sports institutions, YMCA, YWCA, etc. The references listed below also provide excellent information on proper swimming techniques.

Measuring exercise heart rate during a swimming workout is possible, but the validity of the results can be questionable. (Some swimmers leave a watch at one end of the pool and check heart rate after swimming two lengths.) Sports scientists discovered years ago that exercise under water produces a lower heart rate, relative to equivalent exercise on land. Therefore, the swimming heart rate can, at best, be considered a rough guide of exercise intensity. If a new exercise level feels particularly difficult or leaves you tired for the rest of the day, drop back to the previous level for another week.

5-WEEK SWIMMING STARTER PROGRAMME

	Swimming Days per Week	Swimming Time (min.) per session	Swimming Distance (mtr)	Rest time (min.) between Swimming sessions	Repeat Swimming sessions	Total Swimming + Rest time (min.)
1st Week	3	1.5	45	3	2	6
2ndWeek	4	1.5	45	2	3	8.5
3rd Week	4	3.0	90	2	2	8
4th Week	4	5.0	135	1	2	11
5th Week	4	4.5	135	1	2	10

SWIMMING

Level	Distance (m.)	Total Time (min.)
I	270	9
II	270	8
III	360	10
IV	450	13
V	540	15
VI	630	18
VII	720	20
VIII	810	23
Maintenance	900-1350	20-40

MINIMUM PROGRESSION*
(Exercise 3-4 days a week)

Age	Days/Level	Weight kg	Caloric Cost	
			Calories per minute	
			36 m./min.	45 m./min.
Below 30	4	57	8.0	8.9
30-39	6	68	9.7	10.8
40-49	8	80	11.4	12.6
50 and above	11	90	13.1	14.5

Walking

Walking is the number one sport for convenience because it fits nicely into the normal daily routine.

---

* Remember to check your readiness for each new exercise level. See p. 81- 82.

Trips to the corner market and a night or after—dinner stroll, all provide good exercise without a lot of fanfare. Sturdy, comfortable shoes that have good arch support, are the only equipment needed.

The low caloric cost of walking—3-6 Calories per minute, means that exercise duration must be longer than with intensive activity, to expend sufficient energy. Other continuous sports can burn 300 Calories in 30 minutes; with walking, it takes 60-90 minutes. However, you don't have to do it all at once. Separate 15-20 minutes walks throughout the day bring the same results.

Walking is always an excellent exercise for weight control, but the low intensity offers no cardiovascular stimulus for those already in good condition. Walking at 6-7 kmph makes it difficult to elevate your heart rate above the minimum 70% MHR. For this reason, the running programme is generally recommended; but if walking is your 'thing', here are two suggestions for increasing exercise intensity:

1. Find a long, gradually sloping hill to walk up.
2. Carry a small pack on your back and add whatever weight is necessary to keep your exercise heart rate at 70-85% MHR.

There is no starter programme for the Walking Fitness Progression; everyone begins at Level I. Adhere to the listed speeds, distances, and times the best you can. Using a high school track and a watch, you can

WALKING

Level	Distance km.	Speed (kmph)	Total Time (min.)
I	1.0	3.0	20
II	1.5	3.0	30
III	1.5	3.25	28
IV	2.0	3.25	38
V	2.0	3.5	35
VI	2.5	3.5	43
VII	3.0	3.5	50
VIII	3.25	3.5	55
Maintenance	3.5-4.5	3.5	60-80

MINIMUM PROGRESSION*
(Exercise 3-4 days a week)

Age	Exercise Days per Level	Weight kg	Caloric Cost Calories per min. at 3 kmph	3.5 kmph
Below 30	4	57	3.0	3.5
30-39	6	68	3.6	4.2
40-49	8	80	4.2	4.9
50 and above	11	90	4.8	5.6

get a good feeling for the different walking speeds (two laps around the standard track equal 800 metres). You can also plot your own measured distance by driving over the route you select, and checking the distance on the odometer. In addition, you can check

---

* Remember to check your readiness for each new exercise level. See p. 81-82.

your local sporting goods store for pedometers—devices which you can clip to your belt to count footsteps and calculate distance walked. Pedometers cost Rs. 450-600.

Rope Skipping & Stationary Running

Hopping exercises certainly stimulate the cardiovascular system, but they are very hard on the feet, ankles and lower leg muscles. With walking and running, the foot lands—heel first, and the strong, straightened, long leg bones absorb the shock. But during hopping, the ball of the foot takes the initial shock and then transmits the stress to injury-prone ankles and lower leg muscles. This makes hopping exercises very hazardous.

Uncontrollable exercise intensity is another problem with rope skipping and stationary running. (To hop more slowly, you have to jump higher to maintain rhythm; this requires approximately the same energy as short jumps at a quicker pace. So it is very difficult to develop a programme of graduated intensity.)

Therefore, rope skipping and stationary running are not generally recommended. (Competitive athletes may use these exercises for conditioning, but only with a carefully designed programme of interval training: alternate periods of hopping and rest, slowly building up a total workout time of 20-30 minutes).

Stair Climbing & Bench Stepping

Stair climbing and bench stepping are the recommended home exercises for most people. The stress on feet, ankles and knees is greater than with walking, but still well below that of rope skipping and stationary running. Most important, however, the intensity of exercise can be precisely controlled through adjustments in bench height and stepping rate.

Stair climbing can provide adequate exercise with appropriate adjustment of climbing rate to reach the 70-85% MHR training zone. You start with one minute of continual climbing the first week, and add one minute each week thereafter (exercise 3-4 days a week); final maintenance level is 20-30 minutes of continual climbing.

If stairs are not available, a 24-30 cm. stepping bench can be used. If you decide to construct such a bench, be sure it is well made and holds firm even on slippery floors. Follow the progression guidelines for stair climbing. The correct technique involves four steps: left foot up, right foot up, left foot down, right foot down. It's all right to hold on to a nearby rail for balance, but do not pull yourself up on the bench: make the leg muscles perform all the work.

SUMMING UP

Many Sports are excellent for cardiovascular fitness and weight control. Any exercise is beneficial if it produces an exercise heart rate of 70-85% MHR, and expands approximately 300 calories.

Continuous sports like running, cycling, and swimming, which involve continual muscle action, can satisfy the above requirements in 20-30 minutes. The greatest advantage of continuous sports is that exercise intensity can be controlled—slowed down or increased, as the need may be. While selecting a continuous sport is a matter of personal choice, it is imperative that exercise sessions should become a regular habit, 3-4 times a week, year after year.

6

Exercises For Cardiovascular
Fitness: Discontinuous Sports

Most game sports (basketball, racquetball, tennis) are discontinuous. During play, the intensity of exercise varies: one moment you are sprinting for the ball, the next moment you are standing still. Research has shown that you can get fitness benefits from this on-off style of exercise which is comparable to those of continuous sports, providing:

1. There is plenty of vigorous muscular action (exercise heart rate is above 70% MHR for 50-75% of the time);
2. Duration of play is 40-60 minutes; and
3. Frequency of exercise is 3-4 days a week.

Discontinuous sports like bowling and golf do not qualify. Even when they are played vigorously, exercise heart rate rarely exceeds 70% MHR. Baseball is another popular sport that fails the test. Heart rate certainly exceeds 70% MHR when one is running the bases, but this is a miniscule part of the play time.

Several discontinuous sports that do meet the criteria for fitness activities are listed on the following pages. The most popular participant sports—basketball, racquetball and tennis—will be discussed in some detail. Other good discontinuous sports are listed in the Fitness Activities Chart at the end of the chapter.

Fitness is not guaranteed just because you play a recommended sport. You must put enough effort into your chosen sport. Sustained effort generally requires at least a minimal amount of skill. Basic instructions should be the first step in an exercise programme using a discontinuous sport. While you are developing your skill, use one of the continuous sports, like running or cycling, for fitness.

Besides basic skill, exercise intensity generally depends upon two other factors: your opponent's skill level, and whether you are competing or practicing. Two equally skilled players will have the best game, and get the best fitness workout. When one player dominates, playing time diminishes, and neither player gets enough exercise. Competition always increases the tempo of play. Everyone likes to win, and puts in an extra effort.

The next time you play a discontinuous sport, think about these conditions. Try to optimise play intensity by selecting an evenly matched opponent, and play to win!

A few 'spot checks' of heart rate during play will quickly establish your exercise intensity. Make the evaluations immediately after a period of action. If your heart rate is always below 70% MHR, then this game is not for you. By monitoring your exercise heart rate and correlating accompanying physical sensations, you will soon learn what proper intensity (above 70% MHR) feels like. You will no longer need to check your heart rate because you will be a qualified judge of good vigorous exercise. Remember, intensity should be above 70% MHR for at least 50-75% of the playing time.

Basketball

	Caloric Cost—Calories per min			
	57 Kg.	68 Kg.	80 Kg.	90 Kg.
Moderate Play	5.9	7.1	8.4	9.6
Vigorous Play	8.3	8.5	12.2	13.5

Maintenance Level: exercise 3-4 days a week, 30-60 minutes a day.

Vigorous basketball is defined as continuous full-court, five-on-five play. Half-court games are considered moderate intensity basketball. Either way, the energy expenditure is high, and 40 minutes of play will leave most people quite exhausted. It has been said that basketball is a sport for the already fit. You don't play basketball to get into shape; you must be in shape to play it.

The Walk-Jog Starter Programme is a mandatory prerequisite for beginning sport enthusiasts who want to play basketball. Continue with the Running Programme, unless you are able to set up a good game with regularity; running serves as an excellent complementary sport, and it is unusual to be able to find enough players and court time to play basketball 3-4 times a week.

Even with a supplemental running programme, a slow, gradual exposure to basketball play is warranted. Footwork and body moves are very sport specific, and no amount of running can totally prepare your legs for basketball play.

During the first 2-4 weeks, limit your basketball sessions to 20 minutes. Don't get involved in any games; just concentrate on individual moves and shots. If your feet and legs adapt well to this light play, start competing in one-on-one games or half-court play. Keep playing time under 30 minutes; this second month is still a progression phase. By the third month, if all goes well, you should be ready for longer half-court play or short full-court games. This slow conditioning process may seem boring, but not so much if you consider the risks of immediate heavy action—a sprained ankle or torn ligament that will keep you off the court for months, maybe forever.

Basketball players must take special care of their feet and ankles. High-top shoes lend support to the ankles during the rapid stop-start action. Two pairs of socks are advisable, to protect the feet and reduce blisters. *The Foot Book* explains in detail, how to care for your feet and what to do for common problems like blisters and ankle strains.

Racquetball

	Caloric Cost—Calories per min.			
	57 Kg	68 Kg	80 Kg	90 Kg
Vigorous play	8.2	9.9	11.6	13.3

Maintenance Level: exercise 3-4 days a week, 30-60 minutes a day.

Racquetball is a new sport which has found favour among recreational enthusiasts and health professionals alike. Players enjoy the fast-moving action and minimum skill requirement; the simplicity of play allows even novice 'wall-bangers' to experience the thrill of competition.

Health experts recognise racquetball as an excellent sport for cardiovascular fitness and weight control. Energy expenditure during vigorous play is high— more than the required 300 Calories are burned in a normal 40-60 minute game. Three to four days of racquetball each week provides the perfect exercise programme for city people who can't find open spaces for outdoor activities.

The high intensity of racquetball is good for fitness, but it can also be hazardous for sedentary beginners. If you have been inactive for the past six months, complete the Walk-Jog Starter Programme (Chapter 4) before attempting serious racquetball play. Once you begin regular play, keep the intensity of action down the first 1-2 months. The best starting procedure is to reserve a court for yourself and work on skill development for 6-8 exercise sessions. Playing 'cut throat' or doubles will also help reduce initial exercise intensity. If you have to play singles, don't go allout. Pace yourself for the first two months, so your body has time to gradually adapt to the high intensity of competitive racquetball play.

Once you have started a programme of regular racquetball, keep the duration of play down to 30 minutes a day for the first couple of weeks. Make sure there is always a day of rest between exercise sessions. As your fitness improves, extend the exercise time to 40-60 minutes, and play as much as you like. Be ready, however, to cut down playing time if you feel residual fatigue.

In one respect, racquet ball is very similar to basketball: the feet, ankles and knees take a good beating. Again, high-top shoes and two pairs of socks provide protection against sprained ankles and blisters. Most injuries occur when players are tired; either, they play too long at one time or they play day after day without giving their bodies a needed rest.

Tennis

	Caloric Cost—Calories per min.			
	57 Kg	68 Kg	80 Kg	90 Kg
Vigorous Singles	7.0	8.4	9.3	11.4

Maintenance Level: exercise 3-4 days a week, 45-60 mintues a day.

The fitness benefits of tennis are closely related to skill level. The beginner gets little conditioning—and most of that from picking up thousands of missed balls. On the other hand, world class players develop stamina that is comparable to marathon runners. One does not have to play like Jimmy Connors or Bjorn Borg for optimal fitness, but better than average skill is required. In a very general way, one can think of adequate skill as the ability necessary to play respectably in local tournaments. Most people can attain this level of skill over 1-2 years, with basic lessons and regular practice.

As with racquetball, novice tennis players should supplement their developmental programme with other fitness activities. Running is a perfect complementary sport, and it fits nicely into a tennis workout. Thirty minutes of tennis practice, followed by 20 minutes of running, provide both good skill practice and good exercise, all within a reasonable time period. Rope skipping is also a good complementary sport, but you have to be careful about feet and ankle injuries.

Sometimes it is possible for beginners to get a good fitness workout by hitting against a wall or practicing with a ball machine. Periodic checks of exercise heart rate will determine whether these activities are useful for you.

Even with adequate skill there is no guarantee that a tennis match will provide quality exercise. The table of caloric expenditure set out on p. 104, assumes two equally skilled opponents and little or no pauses between games. A match between two players of unequal ability will be less vigorous for both. Some of the loss of exercise can be made up with longer warm-up rallies, with an effort to increase the amount of moderate-intensity exercise. During these rallies, try to keep the ball in play rather than hitting for winners. If possible, work on special drills where one player hits only cross-court shots and the other player hits down the line. After 15-20 minutes of this concentrated play, you can begin the match knowing that no matter how the competition goes, you've had some good exercise.

Doubles tennis is less intense than singles, and exercise heart rate rarely enters the training zone (70-85%MHR). In addition to less general movement, each player receives and serves only half the number of balls he would in a comparable singles match. In defence of doubles, there is evidence that women who play doubles 5-7 days a week have the same fitness levels as women playing a combination of singles and doubles 3-4 days a week. And, of course, there are many older or partially disabled people who can participate in a good doubles match, but, realistically, could never play singles. To summarise, singles is the preferred form of tennis for fitness, but doubles may be of value if it is played vigorously 5 or more days a week.

Fitness Activities

Sport	Caloric Cost—Calories Per Minute			
	57 Kg	68 Kg	80 Kg	90 Kg
Badminton Singles, vigorous	8.2	9.8	11.0	13.0
Canoeing	5.9	7.1	8.3	9.3
Dancing vigorous	5.7	6.9	8.1	9.1
Fencing vigorous	8.6	9.7	11.6	13.6
Handball singles, vigorous	8.2	9.9	11.6	13.0
Horseback Riding trot	5.6	6.8	8.0	9.1
Rowing vigorous	11.4	13.8	16.2	16.7
Skating vigorous	8.6	8.9	12.2	13.4
Skiing downhill	8.1	9.8	11.5	12.6
cross country	9.8	11.8	13.9	15.9
Soccer vigorous	7.5	9.0	10.6	12.2
Squash singles, vigorous	8.2	9.9	11.6	13.0
Water Skiing	6.5	7.9	9.3	10.6

SUMMING UP

Discontinuous sports like basketball, racquetball, and tennis are also beneficial for cardiovascular fitness and weight control. However, since the intensity of exercise varies, as opposed to that continuous sports, the duration of play should be at least, 40-60 minutes to produce a heart rate of over 70% MHR. Certain discontinuous sports like bowling, golf, and baseball, even when played vigorously, rarely exceed 70% MHR.

The debate over the 'best' sport must ultimately revolve around individual preference, because physiological benefits are generally the same, once the general requirements are met. It can be argued that continuous sports are best because of their efficiency. On the other hand, discontinuous sports are favoured by those who enjoy skill development, scoring points and the excitement of competition.

7

Useful Tips For A Healthy Exercise Programme

Up to this point, I have discussed a little of the 'why' of exercise and more about the 'how to'. I have covered the basic informational foundation that all quality exercise programmes are built upon. However, as one becomes involved in regular physical activity, many further questions are bound to arise.

I cannot fully respond to this need without adding several hundred additional pages. Therefore, with some difficulty, I have attempted to select and briefly discuss those topics which seem to be of major interest to exercise enthusiasts. At the end of the book, a comprehensive reference list is offered for those who desire more detailed information.

Keep Your Motivation on A Permanent High

In a way, starting an exercise programme is similar to stopping smoking. Lots of people claim it's easy—after all, they've done it many times before. Health professionals estimate that 30 to 50 per cent of beginning exercisers will drop out within 10 weeks. Obviously, the motivation that initiates exercise tends to fade with time.

But fitness can be maintained only if there is a permanent change in behaviour. We know that the effects of exercise cannot be stored, and benefits are lost as quickly as they were gained. A summer filled with sport and exercise is great, but the fitness will be lost by Christmas without continued regular exercise. Therefore, the secret to a successful programme is lasting motivation. Here are some suggestions that can help you develop lasting motivation:

- ❑ **Look for a small group of friends** to join in your exercise programme. Friends can help in two ways: a scheduled appointment demands a stronger commitment; exercising with friends is more fun. Try to organise a group with more than one person. One friend may get sick or bored or leave town—with three or four friends in your group, hopefully, you can always be assured of a partner. Moreover, with three or four friends, you may get more invitations to exercise; you may have to work to keep your exercising down, rather than fighting to keep it up.

❏ **If you have a preferred sport,** search around for information about tournaments or organised meets. Virtually, every sport you can think of has a local or regional association that offers regular competitive events, at various skill levels. To obtain information, contact sports professionals at the sport clubs, YMCA, YWCA, the 'clubs' listing in the yellow pages or by looking through popular sport magazines. If you have a friend who is deeply involved in a sport, chances are that he already belongs to an athletic association and has information on upcoming events. One competitive event every few months is all it takes to encourage you to keep in shape.

❏ **If your job involves excessive travelling,** it is difficult to maintain a regular exercise programme. The best solution may be an alternative cardiovascular exercise that can be performed within the confines of a motel room. Running in place or jumping rope are possibilities, but remember that stair climbing or bench stepping are the preferred stationary exercises (see page 96). In addition, increasing interest in fitness has led many large hotels to establish internal athletic facilities; others have formed relationships with local clubs in order to accommodate their guests. If you have a choice of where you get to stay when you travel, look for a hotel that offers such facilities.

❏ **Monitoring your vital physical statistics,** and charting the change over time, can provide powerful motivation. Body weight, and waist and hip circumference (particularly in women), decrease over the months with an effective exercise programme. Resting heart rate can be another indication of improving fitness. Before getting out of bed in the morning, check your resting heart rate. Regular exercise will cause a decrease of approximately one beat per minute, every two weeks, for the first 15-20 weeks. After 10 weeks in a programme, it is not unusual to see a resting heart rate change from, say, 60 to 55 beats per minute. You will see even more dramatic changes by checking your exercise heart rate after a measured standard exercise. Stepping up on and then down bench at a standard rate, or running one Km. at a standard pace, are both good tests of cardiovascular fitness. Post-exercise heart rate may drop 10-30 beats per minute over several months of regular exercise. Conversely, if exercise is neglected, both resting and exercise heart rate will begin to speed up to where you started.

Starting Afresh after an Unavoidable Break

Even the most avid sports enthusiast encounters life situations that are incompatible with his exercise programme. Such disrupting experiences as changing jobs, divorce or moving to a new city can easily eliminate motivation for physical activity. Even the good times, like vacations and holidays, can throw you off your schedule. It's best to expect interruptions in your exercise programme.

Getting sick is a special problem for active people. Obviously, any major illness is incompatible with exercise. Your body will certainly tell you when it is time to hang up your shoes, and your doctor will tell you when to resume. During minor illnesses, however, many people wonder whether to continue their exercise programme. As a general rule, it's best to play it conservative and stop all exercise, even if you feel pretty strong. Far too often, the stress of exercise will inhibit your return to health.

Regardless of the type of interruption, restart you exercise programme as soon as possible. The longer you wait, the harder it gets; motivation and fitness tend to disintegrate together.

The re-entry level of exercise depends upon how long you have been inactive. If it's only a week, feel free to pick up where you left off. If 6 months have gone by, then you must start at the beginning again. As a very general rule, figure that, for every two weeks of no exercise, you should drop back one Fitness Progression Level when exercise is resumed. With discontinuous sports games, you should make a conscious effort to keep the intensity of action low for the first one to three weeks.

Selecting the Right Clothes

For most sports, good shoes are the most important item of clothing. They should be the type designed for your sport, and should fit well and feel comfortable. Inexpensive shoes that provide little support or protection can be a major cause of ankle, knee, hip, and back injuries. Buy your athletic shoes from a reputable dealer who is known for high quality shoes.

Socks also provide important protection for the feet. They offer additional cushioning and help protect against the heat of pavement or athletic courts. Two pairs of woollen or cotton socks are recommended, especially for those prone to blisters or athlete's foot.

Your other clothing should be appropriate for the particular sport and environmental condition. Generally, exercise clothing should be light, comfortable and loose fitting. It is better to underdress than overdress because you will soon warm up with physical activity. Avoid tight-fitting clothes that may restrict range of motion, irritate the skin or reduce blood flow.

Wearing rubberised or plastic suits for rapid weight loss is ineffective and dangerous. They only promote water loss through excessive sweating, not reduction in body fat. The water loss will be quickly regained with subsequent fluid intake (and, in fact, you should check your weight after a hot workout and make sure you do replace the lost water). By interrupting sweat evaporation, a rubberised suit forces body temperature to rise higher and higher. If exercise is continued, the temperature regulation system may 'overload', resulting in heat stroke or heat exhaustion.

Don't Punish Your Body

Often, beginning exercisers think they're still back at their high school peak condition, and enter the exercise programme at the wrong level. Even seasoned sport participants can get into trouble when they push for longer distances and faster times. The body has a limit to the amount of exercise it can tolerate. This limit will change with long-term training, but if it is constantly exceeded, general fatigue and tissue damage will result.

If exercise leaves you exhausted, you are, either, playing too long or too hard. Feeling tired and unable to concentrate the rest of the day, are also signs of excessive exercise. (Moderate fatigue immediately after a workout is common, but this should pass quickly.) Actually, proper amounts of physical activity will leave you refreshed and alert. Don't be fooled into thinking that exercise is only doing good when it feels bad. If you notice residual fatigue, reduce the exercise load. Eventually you can build back up, but you must let your body tell you when you are doing too much.

Various muscle and bone injuries also indicate too much exercise—most commonly, muscle soreness, bone bruises, low back pain and shin splints. Rest is the immediate cure, and switching to an alternative sport (like swimming or cycling) will often permit you to maintain fitness while the injury heals. When you return to the original sport, reduce the amount of exercise.

Again, stretching both before and after a workout, as also massage and warm baths, can help prevent muscle soreness. Proper footwear and running on soft surfaces protect against back pain and shin splints. In general, never exercise with pain; rest until the symptoms disappear and then start again at a reduced level.

Eliminate Smoking

Cigarette smoking can effect performance in endurance sports by disrupting the oxygen transport system. Tiny smoke particles irritate the lungs, causing airways to become constricted, and breathing becomes harder because air must be forced through smaller tubes. Changes in airway size occur minutes after smoking begins and can last up to 80 minutes. While resting the change is hardly noticeable, but during exercise, breathing becomes strenuous as insufficient oxygen reaches the bottom part of the lungs. The muscles will tend to tire more quickly as they are served by less blood oxygen.

The carbon monoxide in cigarette smoke compounds the problems of decreased oxygen transport. This small gaseous molecule diffuses quickly into the blood and attaches itself to the same chemical structures that carry oxygen molecules. Unfortunately, carbon monoxide attaches 'better', and the more that is absorbed, the less room there is for oxygen. Again, the problem goes unnoticed during rest because the oxygen demand is relatively small; but even moderate amounts of exercise will seem difficult, because the muscles are demanding a high per cent of the available blood oxygen.

There is never anything good to say about smoking. The risk of lung cancer, heart attack, and chronic obstructive diseases rises with every cigarette. The negative effect on endurance performance is just another good reason for kicking the habit.

All smokers know that cigarettes are unhealthy, but many can not or do not want to stop. It is interesting to note, however, that a very high percentage of sports enthusiasts who used to smoke, give up smoking—apparently the rewards of 'good wind' and increased exercise energy can provide more motivation than the risk of future chronic disease. If you are a smoker, regular exercise may be the best thing you ever did for yourself, in more ways than one.

Exercise to Match Your Age

For the average person, physical regression normally occurs with advancing age: muscular strength and endurance dwindle, and body fat increases. Is this inevitable biologically or simply the result of sedentary living? Research suggests that both factors are involved. There is a natural decrease in fitness over the years, but, it is greatly accelerated in the absence of regular exercise.

Age need not be a barrier to a vigorous lifestyle, so long as you remain active. For example, Clarence de Mar, a famous marathon runner, made it a habit to run twelve miles everyday throughout his life. As a result, he was still competing in 45 km. races up to age 68, i.e. two years before his death (from cancer). Another example was presented in a study by Dr Fred Kasch, an exercise physiologist from San Diego. Dr Kasch examined a group of middle-aged men who ran regularly for 10 years (ages 45-55) and discovered that the mean exercise level and endurance capacity did not change over this period.

So you really do not have to be 'over the hill' after 30. Certainly most of us will never be world class runners like Clarence de Mar, but regular training will provide a level of fitness that will permit vigorous competition, if that's what we want, and, in any event, that will enable us to enjoy life to the fullest. If you have been inactive for years, you cannot expect to regain the strength of youth. Furthermore, as we've pointed out, older people must start at a lower exercise level and progress at a slower rate. But the important point is not how long it takes, but what will be achieved.

Men and Women:
Understanding the Physiological Differences

What are the physical differences between men and women—in terms of strength, stamina, physical conditioning and fitness, and general athletic ability? Up to age 10, there is little difference in body size and physical ability, except for upper body strength. Beyond puberty, however, girls experience, first, a levelling and then, a slow decline in speed, strength, and endurance, whereas, boys continue to improve in all these areas up to age 20-25. These differences in physical capacities are largely attributable to the changes in body composition that occur with maturation. The female, on the average, will be 12 cm. shorter and 18 kg. lighter than the average mature male. More importantly, the female body will have a greater proportion of fat weight (24% fat, for the average college female vs. 15% fat for the average college male) and a lesser proportion of muscle mass. Put another way, if a man and a woman were of equal height and weight, the female would still be at a physiological disadvantage because she would have fewer muscles to move the same body weight.

Will training eliminate these differences between men and women? The gap can be significantly decreased, but, in most cases, physiological equality will never be achieved. Highly active females will have an average body fat of 15-20%, whereas, men will get down to 10-15% body fat with comparable training. Women can improve their endurance capacity dramatically with training, but again, equally trained men will improve 15-30% more. Muscle size and possible muscle strength are related to the level of blood testosterone, the male sex hormone. On the one hand, this means that women can exercise vigorously without fear of developing unsightly muscle bulges. But it also relates to why women cannot achieve the same levels of strength.

Many of the common statistics comparing athletic abilities of men and women can be misleading because the subjects tend to be moderately active males and sedentary females. With a programme of regular exercise, women can effect dramatic changes in body composition, strength, and endurance. At the highly competitive level, men generally have the physiological edge, but at the amateur level, performance differences are often not great.

A Balanced Diet

'You are what you eat' is a common saying, but does it apply to athletic performance? Can the simple ingestion of a particular foodstuff make us run faster, hit a ball harder or jump higher? Can the lack of certain foods impose a negative effect on performance? These questions are very intriguing, and sooner or later, are pondered upon by every competitive athlete. While the 'magic pill' theory will always be tantalising, nutritional experts generally agree that a well-balanced diet is all that is necessary for optimal physical performance.

Without a doubt, protein is the most misunderstood nutrient. Contrary to popular belief, it is not a major source of energy for muscular work. Professional football players do not have to eat steak and eggs for breakfast, lunch and dinner to play their best. Actually, the football player requires no more protein than a sedentary man of equal size. Studies have shown that fat and carbohydrate are more efficient sources of body fuel, and protein is used for energy only when there is an insufficient supply of these other nutrients. Unused protein will be converted to body fat. Protein is certainly required for growth and the maintenance of body tissues, but the optimum amount is much less than most people realise. *Most people take two or three times more than they neeed.*

The use of salt tablets has been advocated for years for exercise under conditions of excessive sweating. While salt depletion is certainly undesirable, it is actually quite rare; the critical loss during most sweat-inducing exercise is water, not salt. It generally takes several days of heavy exercise to deplete salt stores significantly. Generally, the salt in our food more than makes up what is lost. On the other hand, significant amounts of body water can be lost in one to four hours, especially in hot humid climates. We are no longer regular water drinkers, and it can take up to

3 days to replace the amount lost during one heavy exercise session. Competing in a dehydrated condition results in early fatigue and low energy.

To avoid dehydration, drink plenty of fluids before, during and after exercise. You cannot depend on your thirst to let you know when you are dehydrated. Only by checking your weight before and after exercise, will you be able to tell whether you are replacing lost body water.

Your Endurance Potential

After 6-12 months of exercise, many enthusiasts get discouraged because they find they are no longer seeing substantial improvements in their performance. They increase training intensity to the point of exhaustion, and still performance times fall short of expectation. There exists a limit to physical capability, and obviously, some people have greater capacities than others.

Athletic potential is determined by heredity. Most people are simply not born with the physical capacity to achieve world class performances, and no amount of conditioning can alter the fact. It is often said that if a person desires to be a champion athlete, he or she must select the right parents. For example, a large heart is advantageous for endurance events; more blood can be pumped with each beat, allowing greater oxygen transport to the working muscles. Similarly, a preponderance of 'fast twitch' muscle fibres, as opposed to 'slow twitch' muscle fibres, separate the top sprinters and high jumpers from us average people.

Not many people aspire for the Olympics, but we generally hope for, at least, respectable performances relative to our peers. But even at the amateur level, genetic limitations are apparent. People just starting an exercise programme may wonder how much improvement can be made within this genetic limit. One study of identical twin sisters provides some insight. While one sister remained generally inactive, the other became involved in competitive swimming. After a year of constant training, endurance capacity in the athletic sister was 20% higher. In other training studies with adult males, endurance capacity improved 15% on the average, over 4-6 months of training. Those who started out with low levels of endurance improved 20-25%.

It is difficult to estimate individual potential because the possibilities for improvement relate to initial levels of fitness as well as amount of training. In general, however, the normally active adult can expect to improve endurance capacity approximately 20% during a 6-12 month period of regular vigorous activity. Further gains in endurance fitness will be small and earned with great difficulty; the genetic limit will be very near.

SUMMING UP

A healthy exercise programme requires more than just understanding its value and selecting a suitable form of exercise. Sustaining your motivation is a continuous challenge and the real test for a committed exercises. Even if an unavoidable break interrupts your exercise schedule, it is imperative to restart the programme as soon as possible. However, exercise should be resumed at a Lower Progression Level.

While it is essential to remain enthused about exercising, persistent fatique should caution you against over-exercising. People over 30 are advised to maintain a lower exercise rate than their younger counter parts; and women must accept that their pysiological differences, account for them being able to develop less muscular strength than males.

Exercisers should also pay attention to wearing good quality shoes and comfortable clothing— they are essential for body care. Smoking should be eliminated as it hampers the easy movement of oxygen. And finally—a well-balanced diet must go hand in hand with an exercise programme that aims at maintaining a healthy heart.

Glossary

Arm-chair athlete: Knows about a particular subject from what he or she has read or heard about it rather than from practical experience.

Blood pooling: Collection of blood due to its excessive oozing from the capillaries.

Calisthenics: Simple exercises done to keep fit and healthy.

Cardiovascular disease: Disease of the cardia, i.e. heart and vascular, (blood vessels).

Cholesterol: Cholesterol is a white, waxy fat found naturally throughout the body including the blood, and is used to build cells and make hormones. The liver and other organs can manufacture all the cholesterol your body needs. However, cholesterol also comes from the animal foods, such as eggs, meats, butter and whole milk. Cholesterol is not found in plant foods.

Electrocardiogram (ECG): A recording of the electrical activity of the heart on a moving paper strip.

Gallup poll: A survey in which a group of people, specially chosen to represent all the people in a country, are asked for their opinion on a particular topic or subject.

Gerontology: The study of the process of ageing and growing old; how the body undergoes change and the physical problems that old people experience.

HDL: High Density Lipoproteins carries less of the blood's cholesterol. HDL is often called 'good' cholesterol because it appears to carry cholesterol from the lining of the arteries back to the liver for disposal. HDL thus prevents cholesterol from depositing in the arteries, and protects against atherosclerosis and coronary heart disease.

LDL: Low Density Lipoproteins carries most of the cholesterol in the blood. LDL is often called 'bad' cholesterol because high levels of LDL lead to the buildup of cholesterol in the arteries.

Odometer: The instrument that measures the distance travelled by wheeled vehicle.

Orthopaedic injuries: Injuries relating to bone.

Pedometer: A small portable device that records the number of paces walked, and thus, the approximate distance covered. A pedometer is usually attached to the leg or hung at the belt.

Sauna bath: A hot steam bath, often followed by a bath or a swim in cold water.

Ski: One of a pair of long, flat, narrow pieces of wood, metal or plastic that can be fastened to boots, so that the person wearing can move easily on snow.

Softball: A game similar to baseball, played with larger, softer ball.

Stationary bicycles: Bicycles used for exercising in one place.

Steam bath: Immersion of the body in a vessel containing steam. This is done for therapeutic purposes.

Trampoline: Gymnastic apparatus comprising strong cloth held by springs in a large frame above the ground, so that people can do acrobatic jumps and somersaults on it.

Vibrating belts: A device that causes vibration. This is used in massage.

Additional Reading

BOOKS

Vital and Health Statistics of the National Center for Health Statistics, (19), March 16, 1978.

The American Way of Life Need Not Be Hazardous to Your Health by J.W. Farquhar, Stanford: The Portable Stanford, 1978.

The Pipes Fitness Test and Prescription by T.V. Pipes and P.V. Vodak, Los Angeles, J.P. Tarcher, 1978.

How Much Exercise is Enough? by M.L. Pollock, The Physician and Sports Medicine, June 6, 1978.

Athletic Training and Physical Fitness by J.H. Wilmore, Boston: Allyn and Bacon, 1977.

Delong's Guide to Bicycles and Bicycling by Fred Delong, Radner, Pennsylvania: Chilton Book, 1974.

The Complete Book of Bicycling by Eugene A. Sloane, Trident Press, 1970.

The Complete Book of Running by James F. Fix, New York: Random House, 1977.

The Joy of Running by Thaddeus Kostrubala, Philadelphia and New York: J B Lippincott, 1976.

Dr. George Sheehan's Medical Advice for Runners by George Sheehan, Mountain View, California: World Publications, 1978.

The Science of Swimming by James E. Councilman, N.J.: Prentice-Hall, 1968.

Swimming Skills by Frank Ryan, New York: Penguin Books, 1978.

Practical Modern Basketball by John R. Wooden, New York: Ronald Press Co., 1966.

Inside Racquetball by Chuck Leave, Chicago: Contemporary Books, 1973.

The Foot Book by Harry F. Hlavac, Mountain View, California, World Publications, 1977.

Vic Braden's Tennis for the Future by Vic Braden, New York: Little Brown, 1977.

The Inner Game of Tennis by Timothy Gallwey, New York: Random House, 1974.

Textbook of Work Physiology by P.O. Astrand and K. Rodahl, New York: McGraw-Hill.

Physiology of Exercise by H. deVries, Dubuque, Iowa: William C. Brown, 1974.

Handbook for the Young Athlete by R. Gaillard, Palo Alto, California, Bull Publishing Co, 1978.

Nutrition, Weight Control and Exercise by F.I. Katch and W.D. McArdle, Boston: Houghton Miffin, 1977.

Food for Sport by N.J. Smith, Palo Alto, California: Bull Publishing Co., 1976.

Complete Conditioning by D. Shepro and H.G. Knuttgan, Reading, Massachusetts: Addison Wesley, 1976.

You Can Prevent Heart Attack by O.P. Jaggi, Delhi, Orient Paperbacks, 1991.

High Blood Pressure: Causes, Prevention & Treatment by B.K. Mehra, Delhi, Orient Paperbacks, 1988

Yogic Cure for Common Diseases by Phulgenda Sinha, Delhi, Orient Paperbacks, 1976

Yogic Pranayama: Breathing For Long Life & Good Health by K.S. Joshi, Delhi, Orient Paper Backs, 1982

30-Day Cholesterol Program by Barbara Kraus, Delhi, Orient PaperBacks, 1992

ARTICLES

Life Style, Newsweek Magazine, May 23, 1977.

The National Aeronautics and Space Administration-US Public Health. Service Health Evaluation and Enhancement Program by D.C. Durbeck et. al Am J of Cardiology, 30: 784-790 (1972).

Physical Activity and the Prevention of Coronary Heart Disease by S.M. Fox, J.P. Naughton and W.L. Haskell, Ann Clin Res., 3: 404-432 (1971).

Physical Activity as an Index of Heart Attack Risk in College Alumni by R.S. Paffenbarger, A.L.Wing and R.T. Hyde, Am J. Epidemiol, 208:161-175 (1978).

Plasma Lipoprotein Distributions in Male and Female Runners by P.D. Wood et. al, Ann New York Acad Sic 301: 748 -763 (1977).

How Much Exercise is Enough? by M.L. Pollock, The Physician and Sports Medicine, June 6, 1978.

The recommended quantity and quality of exercise for developing and maintaining fitness in healthy adults. Sports Medicine Bulletin, (Position statement by the American College of Sports Medicine) July 13, 1978.